NORA ANSLER

Supplements 101

A Basic Introductory Guide to Supplement, Herb, Mineral, and Vitamin Use

Contents

Introduction 1

1 Chapter 1: Understanding Supplements 3

1.1 What Are Supplements? A Beginner's Guide 3

1.2 The Science Behind Supplements: How Do
They Work? 5

1.3 Types of Supplements: Vitamins, Minerals, and Beyond 6

1.4 The Role of Supplements in Holistic Health 8

1.5 Differentiating Between Natural and Synthetic Supplements 10

1.6 How Supplements Fit Into a Balanced Lifestyle 12

2 Chapter 2: Making Informed Choices 14

2.2 Trusted Brands: How to Choose Reliable Products 17

2.3 Personalized Supplement Plans: Tailoring to
Your Needs 19

2.4 Cost-Effective Supplement Choices Without Compromise 21

2.5 Avoiding Common Marketing Traps in the
Supplement Industry 23

2.6 Building a Basic Supplement Stack for Beginners 25

3 Chapter 3: Safety and Interactions 27

3.2 Side Effects and How to Mitigate Them 29

3.3 Interactions with Medications: What You Need
to Know 31

3.4 Supplements for Pregnant and Nursing Mothers: Special Considerations 33

3.5 Allergies and Sensitivities: Navigating Potential Reactions 35

3.6 Safe Supplement Use: Avoiding Overconsumption 37

4 Chapter 4: Integrating Supplements into Daily Life 39

4.2 Supplements and Meal Timing: Maximizing Absorption 41

4.3 Travel-Friendly Supplements: Staying Healthy on the Go 43

4.4 The Art of "Stacking": Combining Supplements for Greater Effect 45

4.5 Creating a Weekly Supplement Schedule 47

4.6 Supplements and Fitness: Enhancing Performance Naturally 49

5 Chapter 5: Targeted Health Solutions 52

5.2 Managing Stress and Anxiety with Adaptogens 54

5.3 Sleep Support: Supplements for Restful Nights 56

5.4 Digestive Health: Probiotics and Prebiotics Explained 58

5.5 Skin Health: Nourishing from the Inside Out 60

5.6 Immune Boosters: Strengthening Your Body's Defenses 61

6 Chapter 6: Scientific Backing and Emerging Trends 64

6.2 Cutting-Edge Research: What's New in Supplement Science? 67

6.3 Nootropics: Enhancing Cognitive Function Naturally 69

6.4 Anti-Aging and Longevity: Supplements for a Longer Life 71

6.5 The Role of Antioxidants in Health and Wellness 73

6.6 Mindfulness and Supplements: Enhancing Mental Clarity 75

7 Chapter 7: Expert Insights and Real-Life Applications 77

7.2 Case Studies: Real-Life Success Stories in Supplement Use 79

7.3 Understanding the Biohackers: Pioneers in Supplementation 81

7.4 Cultural Perspectives: Global Approaches to Supplement Use 84

7.5 Overcoming Skepticism: Building Trust in Your
Supplement Journey   86
7.6 FAQs: Answering Your Most Pressing Supple-
ment Questions   88
8   Chapter 8: The Future of Supplements   91
8.2 The Role of Technology in Modern Supplementation   93
8.3 Personalized Nutrition: The Future of Supple-
ment Plans   95
8.4 Innovations in Supplement Delivery: Beyond
Pills and Powders   97
8.5 Community and Support: Building a Supple-
ment User Network   99
8.6 Preparing for the Next Wave: Trends to Watch
in Supplementation   101
9   Conclusion   103
Resources   106

Introduction

Years ago, I stood in the middle of a bustling health store, surrounded by rows of colorful bottles and jars. Each label promised miracles—a boost in energy, a sharper mind, a stronger heart. But as I scanned the shelves, a wave of confusion washed over me. What did I really need? What was safe? What was merely a marketing gimmick? Like many, I felt overwhelmed by the choices and the noise surrounding supplements.

This book emerged from that moment of uncertainty, and it aims to be the guide I wish I had back then. "Supplements 101" is designed for beginners, offering a practical pathway into a world of natural healing. It empowers you to use nature's own remedies to enhance your everyday wellness. Through science-backed advice and clear guidance, you will find the tools to integrate supplements into your life with confidence.

Navigating the supplement landscape is not easy. There is a sea of misinformation, safety concerns, and an overwhelming number of options. It's all too easy to feel lost and unsure of where to start. Many people struggle with understanding which supplements are genuinely beneficial and which ones are unnecessary or even harmful. This book addresses these common challenges, providing clarity and direction.

My motivation for writing this book stems from a deep passion for helping others achieve optimal health and vitality. My journey through the confusion of supplement use led me to a place of learning and discovery. I am committed to sharing this knowledge with you, ensuring that you make informed decisions for your health.

The structure of this book is straightforward and user-friendly. We begin by understanding what supplements are and their role in our health. You'll learn how to make informed choices, considering both the benefits and potential risks. We cover safety guidelines, helping you to avoid common pitfalls. Finally, we explore how to integrate these natural remedies into your daily life for maximum benefit.

What sets this book apart is its focus on science-backed information and practical advice; providing a balanced understanding, merging traditional wisdom with modern science. It's about creating a holistic view of health that is both achievable and effective.

As you read through this book, expect to gain confidence in selecting the right supplements for you. You'll understand how to use them safely and effectively, making them a seamless part of your wellness routine. By the end, you will be equipped with the knowledge and tools to take control of your health naturally.

I invite you to engage with this material actively. Explore the chapters, try the recommendations, and see how they fit into your life. This journey is about discovering what works best for you and experiencing the health benefits that nature's medicine can offer. Let this book be your companion as you step into a healthier, more balanced life.

1

Chapter 1: Understanding Supplements

1.1 What Are Supplements? A Beginner's Guide

At its core, a supplement is any product taken orally that contains one or more ingredients intended to add nutritional value to your diet. Supplements come in various forms—think of them as the vitamins, minerals, and herbs you see lining the shelves of health stores. They're not meant to replace a balanced diet, but rather to enhance your nutritional intake, filling in the gaps where your diet may fall short. Whether it's vitamin C for immune support or magnesium for muscle function, these products act as nutritional enhancements, boosting your body's natural capabilities. They are the secret weapon in many people's wellness arsenals, especially when diet alone doesn't meet all nutritional needs.

People often turn to supplements for three main reasons: to fill nutritional gaps, maintain health, and prevent diseases. In our fast-paced lives, it's easy to overlook the importance of a balanced diet. Supplements can bridge that gap, providing nutrients that might be lacking. For instance, those who lack omega-3 fatty acids in their diet, might take fish oil supplements to support heart health. Similarly, those living in northern climates with limited sunlight may supplement with vitamin D to support bone health and immune function. For others, supplements serve as a proactive measure against potential health issues—antioxidants like vitamin E are often used to combat oxidative stress and lower the risk of chronic diseases.

Despite their benefits, supplements are surrounded by misconceptions. Some people believe that taking supplements allows them to neglect healthy eating habits. This couldn't be further from the truth. Supplements should complement, not substitute, a nutritious diet. Another common myth is that all supplements are inherently safe. In reality, taking too much of certain vitamins or minerals can be harmful. It's crucial to follow recommended dosages and consult with healthcare professionals when necessary.

The regulation of supplements adds another layer of complexity. In the United States, the Food and Drug Administration (FDA) oversees dietary supplements under the Dietary Supplement Health and Education Act of 1994. Unlike prescription medications, supplements do not require FDA approval before they hit the market. Instead, manufacturers are responsible for ensuring their products are safe and properly labeled. However, the FDA can intervene if a product is found to be unsafe or mislabeled after it becomes available to consumers. Quality assurance processes, such as third-party testing and certification, help maintain standards, but the responsibility largely falls on the consumer to choose reputable brands.

Understanding supplements means cutting through the noise and focusing on what truly matters—your health and well-being. Armed with the right information, you can make informed choices that support your lifestyle.

1.2 The Science Behind Supplements: How Do They Work?

When you take a supplement, the journey from capsule to cell is a complex dance of biological processes. At the heart of this is absorption, a process that determines how well your body can take in the nutrients you consume. Once you swallow a supplement, it travels to your stomach and intestines, where it's broken down and absorbed into the bloodstream. But absorption is only part of the story. Bioavailability—the proportion of a nutrient that enters circulation and is used by the body—is crucial. Factors like the presence of fat in your meal or even the time of day can significantly impact how much of a supplement your body can utilize. For instance, fat-soluble vitamins like D and E need dietary fat to be absorbed effectively. Once in the bloodstream, nutrients navigate through metabolic pathways, engaging in complex interactions with enzymes and cells to fulfill their roles in maintaining health.

Supplements don't just float around aimlessly; they serve specific physiological functions essential for health. Take calcium, for instance. It's not merely a building block for bones; it plays a vital role in nerve transmission and muscle contraction. Without adequate calcium, your body would struggle to perform even basic tasks. Similarly, omega-3 fatty acids, found abundantly in fish oil, are celebrated for their heart health benefits. They help reduce inflammation, lower triglyceride levels, and even support cognitive function. There's a reason why these nutrients are often recommended by healthcare professionals: their roles are critical, and their impact is profound. Yet, the effectiveness of these supplements isn't just based on anecdotal evidence. Scientific studies lend weight to their use.

The role of supplements extends beyond simple nutritional support; they are potent tools in disease prevention and management. Consider vitamin D, often dubbed the "sunshine vitamin." It's crucial for bone health, yet its influence stretches further, playing a role in reducing the risk of diseases like multiple sclerosis and certain cancers. Similarly, antioxidants like vitamin C and E are known for their ability to neutralize free radicals, potentially lowering the risk of chronic ailments such as heart disease and cancer. These nutrients act as a line of defense, helping the body fend off the damage caused by oxidative stress and inflammation.

Research continues to uncover the depths of how supplements can aid in managing conditions. The evidence is growing, and as it does, so does our understanding of how to use supplements effectively. What remains constant is the potential these small capsules and powders hold. They are not just additions to our diets but powerful allies in our quest for better health, supporting, preventing, and sometimes even healing in ways we are just beginning to understand.

1.3 Types of Supplements: Vitamins, Minerals, and Beyond

Diving into the world of supplements, it's crucial to understand the vast variety on offer. Vitamins, for instance, are often the first to come to mind. These organic compounds are vital for numerous bodily functions. From vitamin A, which aids vision and immune health, to the B-complex vitamins that support energy metabolism and brain function, each plays a distinct role. Vitamin C is famed for its antioxidant properties, while vitamin D is essential for bone health and immune function. These vitamins can be a lifeline when dietary intake is insufficient, helping to maintain the delicate balance of nutrients in your body.

Minerals are equally important, though they often fly under the radar.

Iron, for example, is crucial for forming red blood cells and transporting oxygen throughout the body. Then there's magnesium—essential for over 300 enzyme reactions, including those that regulate blood pressure and glucose levels. Zinc, another mineral, is indispensable for immune function and wound healing. These elements are not produced by the body, so they must be consumed through diet or supplements. They work quietly but effectively, ensuring that the body's myriad processes run smoothly.

Beyond vitamins and minerals, the supplement world offers a treasure trove of herbal and botanical options. Derived from plants, these supplements have been used for centuries in traditional medicine. Ginseng, for instance, is renowned for its ability to boost energy and combat fatigue. Echinacea is a popular choice for immune support, often taken as a preventative measure during cold and flu season. Turmeric, with its active component curcumin, is celebrated for its anti-inflammatory properties, making it a go-to for those looking to soothe joint pain or enhance overall wellness. These botanicals harness the power of nature, offering a more holistic approach to health.

Specialty supplements cater to specific health needs, adding another dimension to your wellness toolkit. Probiotics, for example, introduce beneficial bacteria into the gut, promoting digestive health and enhancing the immune system. These microorganisms are vital for maintaining a balanced microbiome, which is increasingly recognized as crucial for overall health. Adaptogens, like ashwagandha and rhodiola, help the body adapt to stress, supporting resilience and mental clarity. These supplements are tailored to address unique health concerns, providing targeted benefits that go beyond general nutrition.

The form in which a supplement is delivered can significantly affect its efficacy. Capsules and tablets are the most common, offering convenience and ease of use. However, bioavailability—the extent to which the body can absorb a nutrient—can vary between forms.

Liquid extracts, for instance, may offer faster absorption, making them a preferred choice for those seeking quick effects or who have difficulty swallowing pills. Powders provide versatility, allowing users to mix supplements into drinks or food, which can be particularly appealing for those integrating multiple supplements into their routine. Each form has its pros and cons, and the choice often depends on personal preference and specific health goals.

In sum, the landscape of supplements is as diverse as it is complex. With so many options available, understanding the types and forms can empower you to make informed choices that align with your health objectives. Whether you're seeking to fill nutritional gaps, enhance energy, or manage stress, there's a supplement that can meet your needs. Remember, though, that supplements are just one piece of the puzzle; they work best when integrated into a balanced lifestyle that includes a healthy diet, regular exercise, and mindful living.

1.4 The Role of Supplements in Holistic Health

Regular exercise and physical activity are cornerstones of a healthy lifestyle, which offer benefits that range from improved cardiovascular health to enhanced mood and mental alertness. In this context, supplements can play a supporting role. Athletes or fitness enthusiasts might turn to protein powders to aid muscle recovery post-workout, while someone aiming to improve joint flexibility might incorporate glucosamine into their regimen. These supplements don't replace the need for movement but rather amplify its positive effects, helping the body recover, build strength, and maintain flexibility.

Mindfulness and stress management practices, such as meditation or Tai Chi, nurture mental health and emotional resilience. Supplements can support these practices by promoting relaxation and focus. Adaptogens like ashwagandha or rhodiola, for instance, are known for their ability to help the body manage stress, potentially enhancing the calming effects of meditation or yoga. By integrating these supplements, individuals can create a more robust mental wellness routine, fortifying their mind against the pressures of daily life.

The key to effective supplement use lies in balance and moderation. It's easy to be drawn into the allure of adding more and more supplements to one's regimen, but this approach can lead to diminishing returns or even adverse effects. Instead, a thoughtful, balanced approach ensures that supplements complement rather than overwhelm. This means considering one's unique health needs, consulting with healthcare professionals, and adjusting based on personal experiences and outcomes.

Personalization is another critical aspect of integrating supplements into a holistic lifestyle. Each individual's health journey is unique, shaped by personal goals, genetic predispositions, and lifestyle choices. Some may need supplements to address specific health concerns like bone density or cardiovascular health, while others might focus on boosting immunity or improving skin health. By tailoring supplement use to fit personal needs, individuals can create a more effective and satisfying health regimen.

The synergy between supplements and lifestyle changes cannot be overstated. Taking a vitamin D supplement, for example, is more effective when paired with regular outdoor activity, which naturally boosts levels of this crucial nutrient. Similarly, supplements that support sleep, like magnesium or melatonin, work best alongside good sleep hygiene practices. This synergy highlights the interconnectedness of health practices, where each component amplifies the benefits of the others, leading to more substantial, more sustainable wellness outcomes.

1.5 Differentiating Between Natural and Synthetic Supplements

Understanding the distinction between these terms can guide informed decisions. Natural supplements derive their nutrients directly from food sources and plants, undergoing minimal processing. Their production often involves extracting the active components from whole foods, preserving the synergy of nutrients. In contrast, synthetic supplements are crafted in laboratories, where scientists replicate nutrients through chemical processes, aiming to mimic their natural counterparts. This fundamental difference in sourcing and production often dictates their composition and how they interact within the body.

When considering absorption rates, natural supplements generally have an edge due to their complex matrix of nutrients, which can enhance the body's ability to utilize them effectively. Whole-food-based vitamins, for example, often contain co-factors that aid in absorption. Conversely, synthetic supplements sometimes lack these additional components, which can affect how well they are absorbed. However, synthetic options often come with the advantage of precise chemical consistency, ensuring a specific dosage in every serving. Cost is another factor where synthetic supplements often lead, as their mass production tends to be less expensive. This affordability makes them accessible to a broader audience, though some consumers remain wary of their artificial origins. Environmental impact also plays a role in the decision-making process. Natural supplements, when sourced responsibly, can be more eco-friendly, supporting organic farming practices and biodiversity. Synthetic production, while efficient, may involve chemical byproducts that raise environmental concerns.

Consumer preferences often reflect a desire for authenticity and perceived purity, which leads many to gravitate towards natural options.

There's a prevailing belief that natural supplements are safer and more effective, a sentiment rooted in the idea that nutrients from food sources are inherently better recognized by the body. Yet, this isn't always the case, as some synthetic supplements are designed to be bioidentical to their natural counterparts. The perception of natural as superior sometimes overshadows the benefits that synthetic alternatives can offer, such as targeted formulations to address specific deficiencies. This dichotomy highlights the importance of considering individual health needs and goals rather than relying solely on labels.

Choosing between natural and synthetic supplements requires weighing multiple factors, including personal health objectives, budget, and lifestyle values. For some, the decision hinges on the desire to maintain a diet as close to nature as possible, even when supplementing. For others, the assurance of a scientifically validated, consistent dosage might take precedence. It's wise to consult with healthcare professionals who can provide insights tailored to individual needs. Additionally, consumers should research brands and scrutinize labels, looking for third-party testing and certifications that vouch for quality and safety. By understanding the nuances of each type, you can make a decision that aligns with both your health goals and personal beliefs, ensuring that the supplements you choose serve you well.

Reflect and Decide:

Consider your priorities when choosing supplements—are you more concerned with cost, environmental impact, or the natural origin of ingredients? Reflect on your values and health goals to guide your choice.

1.6 How Supplements Fit Into a Balanced Lifestyle

Incorporating supplements into your daily routine can be as straightforward as brushing your teeth. It's about creating habits that integrate seamlessly into your life. Imagine starting your day with a glass of water and a multivitamin. This simple act can set a tone of wellness for the rest of your day, ensuring you kick off with essential nutrients. Morning routines are a perfect time to incorporate supplements that support energy and focus, making it easier to tackle your tasks with vigor and clarity. By aligning supplement intake with the rhythms of your day, you create a nurturing ritual that supports ongoing health.

Meal planning is another key area where supplements can play a role. Consider them an extension of your nutritional strategy. As you plan your meals for the week, think about how supplements can complement your diet. Perhaps you're focusing on boosting your immune system as flu season approaches; adding echinacea or vitamin C to your regimen might be beneficial. Or maybe you're working on muscle recovery post-exercise, in which case protein powders could be added to your post-workout shake. Supplements should enhance your meals, not replace them, ensuring you get the most out of the foods you eat.

When it comes to fitness, supplements can be a game-changer. They can support everything from endurance to recovery. For those who hit the gym regularly, timing is crucial. Supplements like creatine or branched-chain amino acids (BCAAs) can be taken pre- or post-workout to maximize their effects. This integration into your fitness regimen can aid in muscle repair, reduce soreness, and boost performance. Consistency is key here. Just as you wouldn't skip a workout and expect results, supplements require regular use to truly make an impact. Make them a part of your fitness plan, aligning them with your workout schedule for optimal results.

Consistency and routine are fundamental to the effectiveness of supplements. Just as your body thrives on regular sleep and exercise, it responds best to a steady intake of nutrients. This doesn't mean rigidity or inflexibility; it means finding a rhythm that works for you. Maybe it's taking your supplements with breakfast or setting a reminder on your phone. The goal is to make it a natural part of your day, one that requires little thought but delivers significant benefits over time.

Making informed choices is crucial in the supplement world. The market is vast, with countless products vying for your attention. It's important to base your decisions on solid research and align them with your personal health goals. Consider what you are hoping to achieve with supplements and do your homework. Look for reputable brands, read reviews, and perhaps most importantly, consult with healthcare professionals. They can provide guidance tailored to your specific needs and help you avoid any potential interactions with medications or conditions.

To maintain a balanced approach, it's helpful to keep a few practical tips in mind. Start with the basics. Focus on supplements that address your primary health concerns before branching out. Keep track of what you're taking and monitor how you feel. This can help you adjust your regimen as needed. Don't hesitate to make changes; what works well during one season of life may need tweaking in another. Balance is about being adaptable and listening to your body's signals.

As you integrate supplements into your life, remember they are tools to support your health, not quick fixes. They work best as part of a holistic approach that includes healthy eating, regular physical activity, and stress management. By weaving supplements into your daily life with intention and awareness, you create a foundation of wellness that supports your body and mind. This approach empowers you to take control of your health, making thoughtful choices that enhance your well-being every day.

2

Chapter 2: Making Informed Choices

I magine standing in the supplement aisle, rows of neatly stacked bottles stretching endlessly before you. Each promises health benefits, but the labels are a jumble of unfamiliar terms. This scenario is all too common, leaving many of us puzzled and hesitant. Yet, understanding how to decode these labels is key to making informed choices and ensuring that what you put into your body aligns with your health goals.

Supplement labels, by law, include crucial information that helps you make these decisions. At the heart of every label are the active ingredients, which are the substances intended to produce the claimed health benefits. They are the stars of the show, whether it's vitamin C for immune support or magnesium for muscle function. Alongside these are the inactive ingredients, which often serve as fillers, flavorings, or preservatives. Though they don't contribute to the supplement's primary purpose, they play important roles in the product's stability and usability. Understanding these components is crucial, as some individuals may have sensitivities or allergies to certain inactive ingredients.

Daily value percentages on labels provide a snapshot of how each serving contributes to the recommended daily intake of each nutrient.

This information is vital for determining whether a supplement fits your nutritional needs without exceeding safe limits. However, interpreting these percentages requires a nuanced approach, as they are based on general dietary guidelines and may not account for individual differences, such as age, lifestyle, or health conditions. It's important to consider these factors when assessing whether a supplement's daily value aligns with your personal requirements.

Additives and fillers are commonplace in supplements, ensuring product stability and enhancing taste or texture. Binders, for example, help hold tablets together, while preservatives extend shelf life. Yet, not all additives are benign. Some can cause adverse reactions or diminish the effectiveness of active ingredients. Being aware of these potential effects allows you to choose products that align with your health goals and avoid unwanted side effects. Keep an eye out for artificial colors and sweeteners, which may not be necessary and can sometimes have negative health impacts.

Certifications and seals are more than just decorative logos; they signify a level of quality and safety. Third-party organizations, such as NSF and USP, provide these certifications, ensuring that products meet specific standards. NSF Certified for Sport, for instance, guarantees that a supplement has been tested for banned substances and contaminants, while USP Verified indicates that the product contains the ingredients listed on the label in the declared potency and amounts. These seals offer an added layer of assurance, helping you navigate the vast landscape of supplement options with confidence.

When analyzing labels, it's important to adopt a critical eye. Misleading claims can often be found in the fine print, where products might boast about benefits that are either exaggerated or unsupported by evidence. Phrases like "clinically proven" or "miracle cure" should raise red flags, prompting further investigation. Understanding proprietary blends is also crucial. These blends often list ingredients without specifying the exact amounts, making it difficult to assess their true efficacy. Be cautious with products that rely heavily on such blends, as they may not provide the transparency needed for informed decision-making.

Supplement Label Checklist

- **Active Ingredients:** Are they clearly listed, and do they match your health needs?
- **Inactive Ingredients:** Are there any potential allergens or unnecessary additives?
- **Daily Value:** Does the percentage align with your personal dietary requirements?
- **Certifications:** Look for trusted seals like NSF or USP for quality assurance.
- **Claims:** Are the health claims backed by credible evidence or too good to be true?

This checklist can serve as a valuable tool during your next visit to the supplement aisle, empowering you to make choices that truly benefit your health.

2.2 Trusted Brands: How to Choose Reliable Products

In the swirling sea of supplement options, brand reputation stands as a beacon of trust and quality. A brand's reputation is more than just a name; it reflects a company's commitment to safety, efficacy, and transparency. When you choose a supplement from a reputable brand, you are investing in their expertise and their promise to deliver what they claim. This means fewer worries about hidden ingredients or ineffective products. A strong brand reputation often stems from years of consistent quality and positive customer feedback. Trustworthy brands are upfront about their sourcing and manufacturing practices, providing a sense of security that what you're ingesting is both safe and beneficial.

Evaluating a brand's reliability involves a careful look at several key factors. Transparency in sourcing is crucial. Brands that clearly state where they obtain their ingredients and how they process them are more likely to produce high-quality supplements. A good brand will also have rigorous manufacturing practices, adhering to industry standards and often exceeding them. This ensures that each batch meets the highest safety and purity criteria. Customer reviews, while sometimes subjective, can provide valuable insights into a brand's effectiveness and customer service. They offer glimpses into real-world experiences, helping you gauge whether a product might work for you. These reviews often highlight both the strengths and the shortcomings of a supplement, giving you a more rounded perspective.

Among the array of supplement brands, some names consistently rise to the top for their dedication to quality and reliability. Garden of Life is renowned for its organic and whole-food-based supplements, appealing to those who prefer natural options. Thorne Research is celebrated for its research-backed formulations and commitment to rigorous testing, making it a favorite among healthcare professionals. Nature Made is often recognized for its affordability without compromising quality, frequently earning USP verification for many of its products. These brands exemplify what it means to put consumer health first, offering products that are both effective and trustworthy.

While there are many reputable brands, it's important to be vigilant for red flags that may indicate a company is not trustworthy. A glaring lack of contact information should raise concerns—reputable companies should be easy to reach for questions or concerns. Vague ingredient sourcing can also be a warning sign. If a brand does not clearly state where their ingredients come from or how they are processed, it's worth considering other options. These ambiguities can indicate a lack of transparency and potentially lower quality standards. Always be cautious of brands that make grandiose claims without backing them up with credible evidence or certifications. Such claims can often be misleading, aiming to lure consumers with promises that have no scientific grounding.

Navigating the supplement market requires discernment and a willingness to do your homework. By prioritizing brand reputation, examining manufacturing and sourcing practices, and listening to the experiences of other consumers, you can make informed choices that align with your health goals. Recognizing red flags and gravitating towards trusted brands will help ensure that the supplements you choose are safe, effective, and truly beneficial. The peace of mind that comes with knowing you've chosen wisely can make all the difference in your health journey, offering reassurance that you're doing the best for your body and well-being.

2.3 Personalized Supplement Plans: Tailoring to Your Needs

When it comes to supplements, a one-size-fits-all approach rarely meets the mark. Your health needs are as unique as your fingerprint, shaped by your lifestyle, diet, and even genetic makeup. The first step in creating a personalized supplement plan is to assess these individual needs. Start by considering your energy levels. If you often find yourself dragging through the day, it might be time to explore supplements that support energy metabolism. B vitamins, for instance, are crucial in converting food into energy, while coenzyme Q10 is known for its role in cellular energy production. On the other hand, if you find yourself frequently under the weather, immune system support might be a priority. Supplements like vitamin C and zinc are well-regarded for their immune-boosting properties. Taking stock of how you feel on a daily basis can guide you toward the supplements that will best support your health.

Once you've pinpointed your needs, it's time to delve into the tools available for crafting a personalized supplement regimen. Consulting with healthcare providers is a valuable step, as they can offer insights tailored to your health profile. These professionals can help you interpret lab results, recommend specific supplements, and guide you on safe dosages. In addition to in-person consultations, online assessment tools have become increasingly popular. These platforms offer questionnaires that analyze your health goals and suggest supplements based on your responses. While they can't replace professional medical advice, they can provide a helpful starting point for your supplement journey.

With your health needs identified and resources at hand, you can begin crafting a supplement plan. For those looking to reduce stress, consider a regimen that includes adaptogens like ashwagandha, known for its ability to help the body manage stress. Pair this with magnesium, which supports relaxation and sleep, to create a calming routine. If fitness and recovery are your focus, supplements like branched-chain amino acids (BCAAs) or protein powders can aid muscle repair and growth. Omega-3 fatty acids are also beneficial for reducing exercise-induced inflammation. Crafting a plan that aligns with your lifestyle and goals can help you see tangible benefits over time.

As you start implementing your personalized plan, it's important to remember that it's not set in stone. Periodic reevaluation ensures that your supplement regimen continues to meet your evolving health needs. Keep track of any changes in your energy levels, mood, or physical performance. This monitoring allows you to adjust dosages or introduce new supplements as necessary. For example, if you notice improved energy and fewer colds, you might consider maintaining your current regimen. However, if you find that certain supplements aren't delivering the desired effects, it may be time to consult with a healthcare provider for adjustments. This dynamic approach ensures that your supplement plan grows with you, adapting to your changing health landscape.

2.4 Cost-Effective Supplement Choices Without Compromise

Finding affordable supplements without sacrificing quality is a goal many share, especially when navigating the often overwhelming market. One practical strategy is buying in bulk. Purchasing larger quantities can significantly reduce the cost per serving, making it more economical in the long run. This approach is particularly beneficial for supplements you consistently use, like multivitamins or fish oil. It's important, however, to ensure that the products have a reasonable shelf life and that you'll use them before they expire. Another way to save is by keeping an eye out for sales and discounts. Many health stores and online retailers offer periodic promotions, which can substantially cut costs. Signing up for newsletters or loyalty programs often provides early access to these deals, allowing you to stock up when prices drop.

The debate between generic and branded supplements often centers around price and perceived quality. Generic supplements typically offer the same active ingredients as their branded counterparts but at a lower cost. This price difference stems from reduced marketing expenses and packaging costs. However, it's crucial to verify that the generic version meets the same quality standards. Reading reviews and ensuring the product has third-party testing can provide peace of mind. Branded supplements, on the other hand, often come with extensive research and development, offering formulations that might include additional beneficial compounds. While they can be more expensive, the assurance of quality and innovation can justify the price for many. Ultimately, the choice between generic and branded should align with your health priorities and budget constraints.

Prioritizing which supplements to purchase requires a clear understanding of your health goals. Start by identifying the supplements that address your primary needs. If maintaining bone health is critical, calcium and vitamin D should be at the top of your list. For those focused on heart health, omega-3 fatty acids might be non-negotiable. It's easy to get caught up in the allure of numerous supplements, but focusing on those that offer the most significant benefits for your specific situation will ensure your money is well spent. This prioritization not only helps manage costs but also prevents the clutter of unused bottles gathering dust in your cabinet.

Budget-friendly supplementation doesn't mean cutting corners on quality. Instead, it involves being strategic about your choices. Consider integrating nutrient-dense foods into your diet, which can reduce reliance on supplements. Foods like leafy greens, nuts, and seeds are rich in essential vitamins and minerals, potentially decreasing the need for certain supplements. Additionally, combining supplements with a balanced diet enhances their effectiveness, allowing you to purchase fewer products while maintaining optimal health. Another tip is to select multi-purpose supplements. Products that combine several nutrients, like a multivitamin with added probiotics, can address multiple health concerns in one go. This not only simplifies your regimen but also reduces the overall cost.

Remember, maintaining a supplement regimen doesn't have to break the bank. By employing these cost-effective strategies, you can enjoy the benefits of these health aids without financial strain. Consistent evaluation of your needs, coupled with smart purchasing decisions, ensures that your supplement routine remains both effective and affordable, supporting your health goals without compromise.

2.5 Avoiding Common Marketing Traps in the Supplement Industry

In the realm of supplements, marketing strategies can be as enticing as they are misleading. Companies often employ celebrity endorsements to create a sense of trust and allure around their products. Seeing a familiar face promoting a supplement can make it seem more credible or effective. But it's important to remember that these endorsements are often financially motivated and don't always reflect the personal use or genuine belief of the celebrity in question. The health benefits they tout might be exaggerated or even nonexistent. It's crucial to look beyond the star power and scrutinize the actual merits of the product.

Exaggerated health claims are another pervasive tactic. Labels might boast about a supplement's ability to "boost your immune system overnight" or "melt fat away effortlessly." These claims, while appealing, often lack scientific backing. They are crafted to prey on our desire for quick fixes and miraculous results. Such language can be a red flag, signaling that the product's benefits may not be as robust as advertised. Instead of taking these claims at face value, it's wise to delve into the research, or lack thereof, supporting them. Often, you'll find that the promises made are too good to be true, with little scientific evidence to back them up.

Being able to spot misleading claims is an invaluable skill. One common giveaway is the use of terms like "miracle cure" or "revolutionary formula." These phrases are designed to catch your eye and suggest that the product offers something extraordinary. In reality, no supplement can provide a one-stop solution to complex health issues. Another indicator of dubious marketing is the absence of scientific backing. Reputable products are typically supported by research published in peer-reviewed journals. If a company fails to provide evidence or references, it might be wise to steer clear. Look for studies that involve placebo controls and large sample sizes, as these lend credibility to the claims.

Critical thinking is your best ally in navigating the supplement market's maze. Approach each product with a healthy dose of skepticism. Ask yourself whether the claims make sense and whether they align with established scientific knowledge. Consider the motivations behind the marketing—are they genuinely aimed at improving your health, or are they merely trying to sell a product? By analyzing these aspects, you can make more informed decisions. Remember, it's not about being cynical but about being cautious and informed. This mindset will serve you well, not just in selecting supplements but in all health-related decisions.

The history of the supplement industry is littered with marketing failures where bold claims failed to match product efficacy. One notable example is the case of vitamin B17, touted in the 1970s as a cancer cure. Despite its popularity, extensive research debunked these claims, revealing no benefit and potential harm. Yet, for a time, marketing convinced many of its miraculous properties. Similarly, the once-popular ephedra was marketed as a weight loss wonder until it was linked to serious health risks, leading to its ban in many countries. These cases underscore the importance of looking beyond the marketing and investigating the science. They serve as cautionary tales, reminding us that not everything that glitters is gold in the supplement world.

In an industry rife with bold promises, maintaining a critical eye and grounded understanding can protect you from falling prey to marketing traps. The goal is to arm yourself with knowledge, enabling you to distinguish between products that offer genuine benefits and those that ride on the waves of marketing hype. By doing so, you empower yourself to make choices that truly enhance your health and well-being.

2.6 Building a Basic Supplement Stack for Beginners

Starting a supplement stack can feel like assembling a personal toolkit for health, each component carefully chosen to meet your unique needs. The concept of a supplement stack refers to the combination of multiple supplements used together to achieve specific health goals. This approach allows you to target various aspects of wellness simultaneously, potentially enhancing the overall effectiveness of your regimen. For many beginners, the idea of stacking might seem complex, but it's all about simplicity and starting with a foundation that addresses the most common nutritional gaps.

A basic, beginner-friendly stack should cover the essentials—those nutrients that most people benefit from supplementing. A multivitamin is a great starting point. It acts like a nutritional safety net, ensuring you get the vitamins and minerals that your diet may lack. By providing a broad spectrum of nutrients, a multivitamin supports overall health and fills in dietary gaps, making it a practical choice for those new to supplementation. Next, consider omega-3 fatty acids. These essential fats are crucial for heart health, brain function, and reducing inflammation. Many people don't consume enough omega-3-rich foods like fish, making this supplement a valuable addition. Lastly, probiotics are beneficial for maintaining a healthy gut, which is foundational to overall health. They help balance the gut flora, aiding digestion and boosting immunity. Together, these three supplements form a solid stack that supports general health and wellness.

As you become more accustomed to your stack, you might find that your needs change over time. This is where the flexibility of a supplement stack really shines. You can modify what you're taking as your health goals evolve or as new research comes to light. If you start feeling more fatigued, you might add a B-vitamin complex to support energy metabolism. Alternatively, if you're focusing on bone health, adding vitamin D and calcium could be beneficial. The key is to remain observant of how your body responds and to adjust accordingly. It's also wise to stay informed about new findings in nutrition science, as fresh evidence might suggest new supplements worth considering.

Simplicity should always be the guiding principle when building and modifying your stack. It's easy to get carried away with the sheer number of supplements available, but more isn't always better. Starting with a straightforward approach allows you to monitor the effects of each supplement and reduces the risk of interactions or nutrient imbalances. This measured approach ensures that you maintain focus and effectiveness, setting the groundwork for a sustainable routine. As you gain experience and knowledge, your stack can become more tailored, but its foundation should always be rooted in simplicity and necessity.

Remember, the goal of a supplement stack is not to replace a balanced diet but to complement it. Consider your stack as a partner to your lifestyle, enhancing the benefits of healthy eating, regular exercise, and mindful living. By starting with a simple stack and adapting it as needed, you can build a regimen that supports your health journey, adjusting to your life's demands and your body's needs.

In this chapter, we've explored how to make informed choices in the supplement world, from decoding labels to creating a basic stack. This foundation prepares you to navigate the complexities of supplementation confidently. As we look ahead to the next chapter, we will delve into the safety and interactions of supplements, ensuring you have the knowledge to use them wisely and effectively.

3

Chapter 3: Safety and Interactions

Picture this: you're at your favorite coffee shop, sipping a latte while scrolling through your phone. You come across an article praising a new supplement that promises to boost energy and improve focus. Intrigued, you consider adding it to your daily routine. But before you make a purchase, take a moment to consider the importance of dosage—a crucial factor in the world of supplements that determines both their efficacy and safety.

Understanding dosages is like finding the sweet spot between too little and too much. The right dosage ensures that you get the maximum benefit from a supplement without crossing into risky territory. This balance hinges on two key concepts: recommended daily allowances (RDAs) and tolerable upper intake levels (ULs). RDAs represent the average daily intake sufficient to meet the nutritional needs of most healthy individuals. They serve as a guideline for maintaining health and preventing deficiencies. Conversely, ULs denote the maximum daily intake unlikely to cause adverse health effects in the general population. Staying within these boundaries is crucial, as exceeding ULs can lead to toxicity and other health issues. For example, taking too much vitamin A can cause liver damage, while excessive iron can lead to constipation and other complications.

Calculating the appropriate dosage for yourself involves considering a range of factors, including age, weight, and health conditions. Age affects how your body processes nutrients, with younger individuals often requiring different amounts than older adults. Weight and body composition also play a role, as they influence how nutrients are distributed and metabolized. Health conditions can further complicate the picture, as certain illnesses or medications might alter your nutritional needs. For instance, someone with kidney disease might need to limit their intake of certain minerals to prevent further complications. Therefore, it's vital to tailor your supplement regimen to your unique circumstances, rather than relying solely on generic recommendations.

Healthcare professionals are invaluable allies in navigating the complexities of supplement dosages. A consultation with a doctor or nutritionist can provide personalized insights based on your health history and current needs. These experts can help you interpret RDAs and ULs in the context of your life, ensuring that you take the right amount of each supplement. They can also identify potential interactions with medications or other supplements, safeguarding against unforeseen complications. This professional guidance is especially important when starting a new supplement, as it helps establish a safe and effective regimen from the outset.

Individual responses to supplements can vary widely, necessitating adjustments in dosages. Factors such as genetics, lifestyle, and diet can influence how your body reacts to a supplement. For example, one person might experience significant energy boosts from a standard dose of vitamin B12, while another might need more or less to achieve the same effect. It's important to monitor how you feel after starting a supplement and be open to making changes if needed. This might involve increasing the dosage if you're not seeing the desired benefits, or reducing it if you experience side effects. Keeping track of your responses can help you fine-tune your supplement intake, ensuring that it remains aligned with your health goals.

Dosage Reflection Exercise

- **Track Your Intake:** Start a journal to log the supplements you're taking, including dosages and times.
- **Monitor Effects:** Note any changes you observe in your energy, mood, or physical health.
- **Adjust as Needed:** Use your notes to make informed adjustments, consulting with a healthcare provider if necessary.

By understanding the nuances of dosages and using a reflective approach, you can optimize your supplement regimen to support your well-being.

3.2 Side Effects and How to Mitigate Them

Navigating the world of supplements can sometimes feel like walking through a field of potential side effects, where the ground can shift unexpectedly beneath your feet. It's not uncommon to encounter some discomforts as your body adjusts to new substances, and understanding these possible reactions can prepare you for a smoother experience. Among the most frequent side effects is gastrointestinal discomfort, which can manifest as bloating, gas, or upset stomach. This usually occurs when your digestive system rebels against the sudden introduction of a new element. Another common issue is allergic reactions, which can range from mild rashes to more severe symptoms like swelling or difficulty breathing. These reactions remind us that even natural products can cause problems if your immune system perceives an ingredient as a threat.

Mitigating these side effects often hinges on timing and gradual introduction. Taking supplements with meals can significantly reduce gastrointestinal issues. The presence of food helps buffer the stomach lining and facilitates the digestion of the supplement, minimizing irritation. Gradual dosage increments also allow your body to acclimate without overwhelming your system. Start with a lower dosage than recommended and slowly increase it as your body adjusts. This approach helps identify your tolerance level and reduces the likelihood of adverse reactions. Additionally, staying hydrated can aid in digestion and absorption, further easing potential stomach troubles.

Despite these strategies, there are times when side effects persist or escalate, signaling the need for professional advice. Recognizing serious side effects is crucial. Symptoms such as severe abdominal pain, persistent nausea, or any sign of an allergic reaction like hives or difficulty breathing warrant immediate medical attention. These could indicate that a supplement is not compatible with your body or that an interaction with other medications or conditions is occurring. Consulting a healthcare provider can prevent minor issues from becoming significant health concerns. They can offer insights into whether you should continue with the supplement, adjust the dosage, or explore alternative options.

Monitoring your body's response to supplements is essential for maintaining your health and safety. Keeping a side effects checklist can be immensely helpful. Note the supplement name, dosage, and any side effects you experience, along with their duration and intensity. This practice not only helps you track patterns but also provides valuable information to share with your healthcare provider. A detailed record can facilitate more informed discussions and lead to tailored advice that aligns with your unique health profile. Regularly reviewing this checklist empowers you to make proactive decisions about your supplement regimen, fostering a safer and more effective experience.

3.3 Interactions with Medications: What You Need to Know

Imagine you're taking a stroll through your local pharmacy, a prescription in hand. As you pick up your medication, a colorful bottle of supplements catches your eye, promising benefits that align perfectly with your health goals. However, what many don't realize is that combining supplements with medications isn't always straightforward. Supplements can interact with drugs in ways that alter their effectiveness or increase the risk of side effects. For instance, vitamin K, known for its role in blood clotting, can interfere with blood thinners like warfarin. This interaction can negate the medication's effects, leading to potentially dangerous clotting issues.

Another common interaction involves calcium supplements and thyroid medications. Calcium can bind with thyroid hormones, preventing proper absorption. This means the medication might not work as intended, leaving thyroid levels unbalanced. Such interactions highlight the importance of timing and dosing, ensuring that both supplements and medications work harmoniously. These examples underscore a critical point: supplements, despite their natural image, can have potent effects on how medications function within your body.

To safely navigate the complex landscape of supplement-drug interactions, it's vital to assess the risks. Start by reviewing your medication profiles. This involves understanding the purpose of each medication you're taking and the potential interactions listed by the manufacturer. Many pharmacists provide detailed information about possible interactions, which can serve as a valuable resource. Consulting a pharmacist is a proactive step that can prevent adverse effects. These professionals can offer insights into how different substances might interact and suggest strategies to mitigate risks.

Some supplements are notorious for their interactions with medications. St. John's Wort, often used for mood support, can significantly affect the metabolism of various drugs. It can reduce the effectiveness of antidepressants, birth control pills, and even some heart medications. Ginkgo Biloba, another popular supplement, is known for its potential to thin the blood. When taken alongside anticoagulants, it can increase the risk of bleeding. These examples illustrate why it's crucial to approach supplement use with a sense of caution and awareness.

Involving healthcare providers in your supplement decisions is not just a recommendation—it's a necessity. Doctors and pharmacists can provide guidance tailored to your unique health profile, considering both current medications and overall health goals. They can help identify potential interactions before they become problems, offering alternatives or adjustments to ensure safety. While supplements can offer numerous health benefits, their integration with medications requires careful consideration and professional oversight. By engaging with healthcare professionals, you ensure that your approach to supplements supports rather than hinders your health journey.

3.4 Supplements for Pregnant and Nursing Mothers: Special Considerations

Pregnancy and nursing are unique stages in life that demand special attention to nutrition. As your body works harder to support both you and your baby, the need for certain nutrients becomes more pronounced. Iron, for example, is crucial during pregnancy due to the increased blood volume required to support your growing baby and placenta. Iron helps in the production of hemoglobin, which carries oxygen to your tissues and your baby. A deficiency can lead to anemia, a condition that can cause fatigue and complications during delivery. Alongside iron, folate is another vital nutrient that plays a significant role in preventing neural tube defects in the developing fetus. These defects can affect the brain and spinal cord, so ensuring adequate folate intake is key during the early stages of pregnancy. Omega-3 fatty acids are equally important, contributing to the development of your baby's brain and eyes. These can be found in fish oil or algae-based supplements, offering a plant-based alternative for those who prefer it.

While the nutritional needs during these stages are unique, safe supplementation practices can help meet them effectively. Prenatal vitamins are designed to provide a broad spectrum of nutrients tailored for pregnancy, including the appropriate levels of iron and folate. They serve as a convenient way to ensure you and your baby receive necessary nutrients even when dietary intake may fall short. Calcium and Vitamin D are also important, supporting bone health for both you and your baby. Adequate intake helps prevent the depletion of your bone mass, as the developing fetus requires a steady supply of these nutrients. These supplements work best in conjunction with a balanced diet rich in whole foods, offering a comprehensive approach to nutrition during pregnancy and nursing. However, it's important to remember that supplements are meant to complement—not replace—a healthy diet.

While many supplements can offer benefits, some should be avoided during pregnancy and nursing due to potential risks. High-dose vitamin A, for instance, can lead to developmental abnormalities in the fetus when consumed in excess. It's crucial to monitor intake and ensure it doesn't exceed the recommended daily allowance. Certain herbal remedies, such as black cohosh and goldenseal, may pose risks as well, potentially leading to complications like premature labor or miscarriage. Always exercise caution with herbal supplements, as they can have powerful effects that are not suitable for pregnant or nursing mothers. Additionally, some supplements might not be well-studied in pregnant populations, so their safety profiles remain uncertain.

The importance of consulting healthcare providers cannot be overstated, especially during pregnancy and nursing. Your doctor or midwife can offer personalized advice based on your health history and nutritional needs, ensuring that any supplementation aligns with your specific circumstances. They can help identify safe options and recommend appropriate dosages, minimizing risks to you and your baby. Regular check-ups provide an opportunity to discuss any concerns or symptoms you may experience, allowing for timely adjustments to your supplementation plan if needed. This professional guidance is invaluable, providing peace of mind and supporting the health of both you and your child.

3.5 Allergies and Sensitivities: Navigating Potential Reactions

Imagine standing in the supplement aisle, eager to boost your health, only to realize the daunting task of finding products that won't trigger an allergic reaction. Allergies in supplements are more common than one might think, especially when you consider the wide array of ingredients used. For instance, gluten and lactose often find their way into supplements as fillers or binders, posing a problem for those with sensitivities or intolerances. Similarly, glucosamine, a popular supplement for joint health, is often derived from shellfish, making it a potential allergen for individuals with shellfish allergies. Identifying these allergens is the first step in making safe choices.

Managing these sensitivities requires diligence and a bit of detective work. The most effective strategy is to read ingredient labels thoroughly. This might seem straightforward, but it involves more than just a cursory glance. Look for hidden sources of common allergens, which can be listed under various names. Gluten, for instance, might be labeled as maltodextrin or dextrin, while lactose could appear as whey or casein. Familiarizing yourself with these terms can prevent accidental exposure. Additionally, seeking hypoallergenic products can offer peace of mind. These are specifically formulated to minimize the risk of allergic reactions, often using alternative ingredients that serve the same purpose without the associated risks.

Another layer of protection in navigating supplement allergies is allergy testing and consultations. If you're unsure about potential sensitivities, undergoing allergy testing can provide clarity. These tests can identify specific allergens your body reacts to, guiding your supplement choices. Consulting with an allergist or healthcare provider can offer personalized advice and help you develop a plan that ensures safety. They can also recommend alternatives or safer formulations that align with your health needs. This proactive approach not only protects you but also empowers you to make informed decisions about your health.

Consider the story of Emily, a young professional who struggled with persistent stomach discomfort after starting a new multivitamin. Suspecting an allergy, she meticulously reviewed the ingredients and realized that lactose was listed as a filler. Being lactose intolerant, Emily switched to a lactose-free version and found immediate relief. This experience taught her the value of being vigilant about ingredient labels and seeking products that cater to her specific needs. Her journey highlights the importance of being proactive and informed, turning a potentially frustrating situation into an opportunity for learning and growth.

Managing allergies and sensitivities in supplements is about being informed and cautious. By understanding common allergens, diligently reading labels, and seeking professional guidance when necessary, you can navigate the supplement world with confidence. This approach ensures that you reap the benefits of supplementation without compromising your health.

3.6 Safe Supplement Use: Avoiding Overconsumption

In the world of supplements, more isn't always better. Overconsumption poses significant risks, transforming beneficial nutrients into potential hazards. When you take too much of a supplement, the body can experience toxicity, a state where excessive amounts of a nutrient accumulate to harmful levels. This can manifest as nausea, headaches, or even more severe symptoms like liver damage in the case of excessive vitamin A or iron intake. Long-term health risks lurk when overconsumption persists, potentially leading to chronic conditions or exacerbating existing health issues. For instance, an overload of calcium supplements may contribute to kidney stones or cardiovascular problems. Recognizing these risks is key to using supplements safely and effectively.

To prevent overconsumption, it's crucial to adhere to recommended dosages. These guidelines are not mere suggestions but carefully calculated limits based on research and established daily needs. Avoiding redundant supplements is another practical step. Sometimes, multiple products can contain overlapping ingredients, leading to unintended excessive intake. For example, if you're already taking a multivitamin, adding individual vitamin tablets might push your intake beyond safe levels. By reviewing the contents of each supplement, you can streamline your regimen, ensuring you only take what's necessary. This not only minimizes the risk of overconsumption but also simplifies your routine, making it easier to stick to consistently.

Routine check-ups play a vital role in maintaining a balanced supplement regimen. Regular health assessments allow you to monitor how supplements are impacting your body and adjust your intake accordingly. Blood tests can reveal nutrient levels, highlighting any deficiencies or excesses. These check-ups provide an opportunity to discuss your supplement use with healthcare professionals, who can offer tailored advice and help recalibrate your dosages if needed. This proactive approach ensures that you're not only meeting your nutritional needs but doing so safely. It's a way to keep your health in check, using supplements as a supportive tool rather than a crutch.

Recognizing signs of overconsumption is crucial for making timely adjustments. Symptoms like persistent fatigue, digestive issues, or unusual changes in mood or energy levels can indicate that your body is receiving too much of a certain nutrient. If you suspect overuse, the first step is to reassess your supplement intake. Consider reducing or temporarily pausing certain supplements to see if symptoms improve. Consulting with a healthcare provider can provide clarity, helping to identify which supplements might be the culprits. By staying attuned to your body's signals, you can make informed decisions that keep your supplement routine both effective and safe.

As you navigate the balance of supplementation, remember that awareness and moderation are your best allies. Supplements hold the potential to enhance health when used thoughtfully, complementing a balanced diet and lifestyle. But like any powerful tool, they require respect and understanding to wield effectively. With the insights from this chapter, you are equipped to make informed choices, avoiding the pitfalls of overconsumption while reaping the benefits supplements can offer.

As we close this chapter, remember the importance of using supplements wisely, respecting their power to both help and harm. With this foundation, you're ready to explore the next chapter, where we'll dive into integrating these natural allies into your daily routine with balance and purpose, enhancing your journey toward optimal health.

4

Chapter 4: Integrating Supplements into Daily Life

Imagine the sun rising, casting a warm glow over your room, as you shake off the remnants of sleep. You head to the kitchen and open the cabinet, reaching for a small bottle that starts your day on a positive note. This simple act of taking supplements can transform your morning into a moment of empowerment, setting the stage for the day ahead. A morning supplement routine can be a powerful ritual, providing your body with the nutrients needed to kickstart energy levels and elevate mood.

B vitamins are a prime example of energy-boosting supplements that can make a world of difference when taken in the morning. Known for their role in converting food into energy, these vitamins support cellular processes that keep you alert and focused throughout the day. Whether you're facing a long day at work or a busy schedule of classes, starting with B vitamins might just give you the extra push you need. Similarly, omega-3 fatty acids, often found in fish oil, are recognized for their mood-enhancing properties. These essential nutrients help maintain brain health, potentially improving mental clarity and reducing feelings of stress and anxiety. By incorporating omega-3s into your morning routine, you can set a positive tone mentally and emotionally, preparing you to tackle the day's challenges.

Establishing a consistent morning routine for supplements is key to reaping their full benefits. Like any healthy habit, it requires intention and a bit of planning. Setting reminders can be a simple yet effective way to ensure you don't forget your daily dose. Whether it's a phone alarm or a sticky note on your fridge, these prompts can make all the difference. Pairing your supplements with your morning beverage—be it coffee, tea, or a smoothie—can also help integrate this habit seamlessly into your routine. As you sip your drink, you can easily take your supplements, reducing the likelihood of skipping them amidst the morning rush.

Certain supplements are particularly effective when taken in the morning. Probiotics, for instance, are best consumed on an empty stomach, as this timing can enhance their ability to colonize the gut and promote digestive health. Starting your day with probiotics can pave the way for improved digestion and a balanced gut microbiome, which is crucial for overall well-being. Antioxidants like vitamin C are another morning staple, offering protection against oxidative stress and supporting immune function. By taking them early, you provide your body with a defense mechanism that prepares you for potential environmental stressors encountered throughout the day.

Consider the experience of Alex, a young professional who struggled with energy slumps and a lack of focus. He decided to revamp his morning routine by incorporating a B-complex vitamin and omega-3 supplement alongside his breakfast. Within weeks, Alex noticed a significant improvement in his energy levels and mental clarity, allowing him to excel at work and maintain a positive mood. This simple change not only transformed his mornings but also set a tone of productivity and well-being for his entire day. Similarly, Sarah, a student, found relief from digestive issues by taking probiotics each morning. This adjustment helped her maintain a balanced gut health, reducing discomfort and allowing her to focus better on her studies.

These examples illustrate how a thoughtful approach to morning supplements can enhance your daily life. By choosing the right supplements and integrating them into a consistent routine, you can support your body's needs and promote a sense of balance and vitality. The morning is a fresh start, an opportunity to nourish your body and mind, setting a foundation for a day filled with energy and positivity.

Morning Supplement Checklist

- **Energy Boost:** Consider B vitamins for converting food into energy.
- **Mood Enhancement:** Omega-3s can support brain health and reduce stress.
- **Digestive Support:** Probiotics taken on an empty stomach enhance gut health.
- **Immune Protection:** Start the day with antioxidants like vitamin C.

4.2 Supplements and Meal Timing: Maximizing Absorption

Timing is everything when it comes to supplements. How and when you take them can significantly influence their effectiveness. Consider fat-soluble vitamins like A, D, E, and K. These vitamins require dietary fat for proper absorption, making them ideal companions to meals that include healthy fats. Imagine a breakfast of avocado on whole-grain toast or a salad drizzled with olive oil at lunch. These meals provide the necessary fats to help your body absorb these vital nutrients more efficiently. On the other hand, water-soluble vitamins, such as vitamin C and the B vitamins, are best taken on an empty stomach. Consuming them with a glass of water before breakfast can enhance their absorption, as they dissolve quickly in water and are absorbed directly into the bloodstream.

Pairing supplements with meals isn't just about absorption; it's also about maximizing the benefits they offer. Calcium, for instance, is best taken with meals, as food stimulates the production of stomach acid, which aids in calcium absorption. Including calcium-rich foods like yogurt or leafy greens in your meal can create an environment conducive to better absorption. In contrast, iron supplements should be taken between meals. Foods high in calcium, such as dairy, can interfere with the absorption of iron. To avoid this, consider taking your iron supplement with a source of vitamin C, like a glass of orange juice, which can enhance iron absorption. This strategic pairing ensures that each supplement works to its full potential, supporting your health goals effectively.

Not all foods play nicely with supplements, and being aware of these interactions can prevent potential hiccups in your regimen. Certain foods can inhibit the absorption of specific nutrients, undermining the effectiveness of your supplements. For example, the tannins in tea and coffee can interfere with iron absorption, so it's wise to avoid these beverages around the time you take your iron supplement. Similarly, high calcium foods can impede the absorption of zinc and magnesium if taken simultaneously. Understanding these interactions allows you to plan your meals and supplement intake strategically, ensuring you get the most out of every dose.

To illustrate how you might organize your day, consider this sample schedule: Start your morning with a glass of water and your water-soluble vitamins, ensuring an empty stomach enhances their absorption. With breakfast, including healthy fats, take your multivitamin and omega-3 supplement. Mid-morning is an excellent time for your iron supplement, paired with a vitamin C-rich snack like an orange. Enjoy lunch with a calcium-rich food and take your calcium supplement to support bone health. This structure not only optimizes absorption but also creates a routine that becomes second nature over time, seamlessly integrating into your daily life. By aligning your supplement intake with your meals, you can maximize their benefits and support your well-being effectively.

Throughout the day, pay attention to how your body responds to this regimen. Adjusting the timing based on how you feel can be an invaluable part of making your routine work for you. The goal is to find a balance that fits your lifestyle while ensuring your body receives the nutrients it needs to function optimally. This approach transforms supplements from mere additions to our diet into integral parts of a daily routine that supports health and vitality. Through thoughtful timing and mindful eating, your supplements can become powerful allies in your quest for wellness.

4.3 Travel-Friendly Supplements: Staying Healthy on the Go

Traveling introduces a unique set of challenges when it comes to maintaining a consistent supplement routine. The hustle of airports, the excitement of new destinations, and the change in daily rhythms can all conspire to throw you off track. However, with a bit of planning, it's entirely possible to keep your health goals in sight while on the move. First, consider the types of supplements that travel well. Multivitamin packs are a convenient choice, offering a compact solution that covers a broad spectrum of nutrients in individually wrapped servings. These packs take up minimal space and are easy to toss into your bag. Another excellent option is probiotic capsules, which support digestive health—a crucial factor when experiencing new cuisines and water sources that your system isn't accustomed to. These capsules are typically shelf-stable, making them ideal for travel without the need for refrigeration.

Maintaining your supplement routine on the road requires organization and foresight. Using a pill organizer can be a lifesaver, especially for longer trips. These handy tools allow you to pre-package doses according to your travel schedule, ensuring you never miss a beat. They're especially useful if you're juggling multiple supplements and need to keep track of what to take each day. Another tip is to integrate your supplements into your daily travel routine, perhaps taking them with breakfast or before heading out for the day. This consistency mirrors your home routine, making it easier to remember and stick to your regimen. Pre-packaging doses in small, resealable bags is another effective method, particularly for shorter trips or when space is at a premium. This approach minimizes bulk and ensures you carry only what you need.

Traveling with supplements involves navigating a few regulatory hurdles, particularly when flying. The Transportation Security Administration (TSA) permits supplements in both carry-on and checked luggage, but it's wise to keep them in their original packaging for easy identification. This can help avoid any confusion or delays at security checkpoints. When traveling internationally, customs regulations may vary, so it's crucial to research the destination country's rules regarding supplements. Some countries have restrictions on certain ingredients or require documentation, such as a doctor's note or prescription, to bring supplements into the country. Being informed and prepared ensures a smooth transition through customs and keeps your supplements safe.

Consider the story of Jake, an avid traveler who frequently journeys for work. On a recent trip to Europe, he relied on multivitamin packs and probiotic capsules to support his immune system and digestive health. By pre-packaging his supplements in a compact pill organizer,

Jake maintained his routine effortlessly, despite the time zone changes and hectic schedule. This simple preparation allowed him to focus on his meetings and enjoy his travels, knowing his health was well-supported. Similarly, Emily, who backpacked through Southeast Asia, found that carrying her supplements in resealable bags minimized space and weight in her backpack. She consulted the customs regulations of each country she visited, ensuring compliance and avoiding any issues at border crossings.

These anecdotes highlight the importance of preparation and adaptability when it comes to traveling with supplements. By choosing portable options, organizing your doses, and understanding regulatory requirements, you can maintain your health regimen no matter where your travels take you. The key is to integrate these practices into your travel plans, ensuring that your supplements are as much a part of your journey as your passport and itinerary.

4.4 The Art of "Stacking": Combining Supplements for Greater Effect

Imagine piecing together a puzzle where each piece enhances the others, creating a picture of complete health. This is the essence of supplement stacking—combining specific nutrients to amplify their benefits. When done thoughtfully, stacking can address multiple health goals simultaneously, offering a well-rounded approach to wellness. Consider the concept of complementary nutrient combinations. Certain vitamins and minerals work synergistically, meaning they enhance each other's absorption or effectiveness. For instance, vitamin D can improve calcium absorption, making a stack of these nutrients beneficial for bone health. Enhanced bioavailability is another advantage, where the presence of one nutrient increases the body's ability to absorb another, maximizing the impact of your supplements.

An effective stack is like a recipe for success, tailored to specific health goals. Take the joint support stack, for example. It combines glucosamine, chondroitin, and MSM (methylsulfonylmethane). These ingredients work together to support joint health by reducing inflammation and promoting cartilage repair. Glucosamine and chondroitin are known for their role in maintaining cartilage structure, while MSM provides sulfur, a key component in joint health. Together, they create a powerful trio that can help alleviate joint discomfort and improve mobility. Another popular combination is the immune support stack, featuring vitamin C, zinc, and echinacea. Vitamin C is a well-known antioxidant, protecting cells from damage and boosting immune function. Zinc plays a critical role in immune cell development, while echinacea is often used to reduce the duration of colds. This stack bolsters the immune system, making it a go-to during flu season or times of increased stress.

While stacking can offer numerous benefits, it's crucial to approach it with caution. Avoiding redundant nutrients is a primary consideration. Overlapping ingredients can lead to excessive intake, potentially causing adverse effects. For instance, taking multiple supplements containing high levels of vitamin A can lead to toxicity, affecting liver health. Monitoring cumulative dosages ensures that you're not exceeding recommended limits, maintaining the balance necessary for safe supplementation. Keeping track of your stack components and their dosages helps prevent unintended excess. It's also wise to consult with healthcare professionals, who can provide guidance on safe stacking practices tailored to your health profile.

Expert opinions shed light on the best practices for stacking supplements. Nutritionists often emphasize the importance of understanding the interactions between different nutrients. Some combinations can inhibit absorption, negating the benefits you hope to achieve. For example, calcium can interfere with the absorption of iron, so they should be taken at different times of the day. Nutritionists also recommend starting with a basic stack and gradually adding components as needed. This approach allows you to observe how your body responds, making adjustments based on real-world feedback. Consulting with experts can provide personalized insights, ensuring your stack aligns with your health goals and lifestyle.

Incorporating stacking into your routine doesn't have to be complicated. Start by identifying your primary health objectives, whether it's boosting immunity, supporting joint health, or enhancing energy levels. From there, select nutrients that work well together, creating a stack that targets your specific needs. It's about finding the right balance, where each supplement complements the others, enhancing the overall effect. As you experiment with stacking, pay attention to how your body responds, making adjustments to optimize your regimen. This personalized approach ensures that your supplements work in harmony, supporting your path to better health.

4.5 Creating a Weekly Supplement Schedule

Incorporating supplements into your lifestyle can feel daunting without a clear plan. Crafting a weekly supplement schedule can streamline this process, ensuring consistency and effectiveness. The idea is to rotate supplements and schedule rest days, creating a balanced routine that aligns with your health goals. Rotating supplements prevents your body from becoming too accustomed to a particular nutrient, which can sometimes diminish its effectiveness over time. For instance, you might take a higher-dose vitamin C supplement three times a week, allowing your body to utilize it more efficiently without overwhelming your system. Meanwhile, rest days provide your body with a break, allowing it to reset and ensuring that you're not overloading your system with unnecessary nutrients.

A structured schedule also serves as a powerful tool in reducing forgetfulness, a common hurdle for many. By having a clear plan laid out, you can easily track which supplements to take on specific days, minimizing the chances of missing a dose. Moreover, a well-organized schedule makes it easier to monitor the effects of each supplement. You can note any changes in energy levels, mood, or overall health, attributing them to the specific supplements taken. This tracking allows for adjustments, ensuring that your regimen remains effective and tailored to your needs. The benefits extend beyond mere organization; they foster a sense of discipline and routine, essential components for achieving long-term health benefits.

To help you get started, consider using a weekly supplement planner. Imagine a simple chart where each day of the week is divided into sections—morning, afternoon, and evening. In each section, you list the supplements you plan to take, along with the dosage. This visual aid acts as a daily reminder, making it easier to incorporate supplements into your routine. You might find it helpful to color-code different types of supplements, such as vitamins, minerals, and probiotics, to quickly identify what you need to take. This planner becomes a personalized guide, one you can tweak as your needs evolve.

The success of a structured supplement schedule is evident in the experiences of many who have embraced this approach. Take Maria, for example, who struggled with maintaining a consistent intake of her supplements due to a busy work schedule. By implementing a weekly planner, she found it easier to remember her supplements and noticed an improvement in her energy levels and focus. Similarly, Tom, who initially felt overwhelmed by the variety of supplements he was taking, streamlined his regimen using a planner. This allowed him to track which supplements delivered tangible benefits and which ones were unnecessary. Both Maria and Tom credit their structured approach to the significant improvements they've seen in their health, demonstrating the effectiveness of planning.

Organizing your supplement schedule might seem like a task, but it becomes second nature with practice. Consider starting with a simple setup, focusing on your core supplements and gradually incorporating new ones as needed. Pay attention to how your body responds and be open to making adjustments. The goal is to create a schedule that fits seamlessly into your life, supporting your health goals without adding stress. This methodical approach not only enhances the efficacy of your supplements but also empowers you to take control of your health in a manageable way. By dedicating a small amount of time each week to planning, you can reap the rewards of a thoughtful, well-organized supplement routine that supports your overall well-being.

4.6 Supplements and Fitness: Enhancing Performance Naturally

In the realm of fitness, supplements serve as potent allies, lending a hand where diet and exercise might fall short. Consider protein supplements. They are a staple for athletes aiming to enhance muscle recovery. After a vigorous workout, your muscles need to repair and grow stronger. Protein provides the building blocks, or amino acids, necessary for this process. Whether you opt for whey, soy, or a plant-based blend, the right protein supplement can make a significant difference in how quickly and effectively your muscles recover, allowing you to push harder in future workouts. Alongside protein, creatine is another powerhouse supplement known for boosting strength and endurance. It helps replenish ATP, the energy currency of cells, which can enhance performance during high-intensity activities. Creatine has been studied extensively and is recognized for its role in increasing muscle mass and improving athletic performance, particularly in activities like weightlifting and sprinting.

Aligning supplements with your workout schedule is crucial for maximizing their benefits. Pre-workout supplements often include ingredients like caffeine or beta-alanine, which prepare your muscles for exertion and boost energy levels. Taking them about 30 minutes before exercise can optimize performance. On the flip side, post-workout recovery aids focus on replenishing glycogen stores and supporting muscle repair. Supplements like branched-chain amino acids (BCAAs) and protein shakes are ideal post-exercise, helping to reduce muscle soreness and accelerate recovery. Timing is key, as consuming these nutrients soon after your workout capitalizes on the body's increased ability to absorb them. This strategic approach ensures that your body receives the support it needs at the right moments, enhancing overall fitness outcomes.

Hydration plays a pivotal role in the efficacy of supplements, especially during intense exercise. Your body loses fluids and electrolytes through sweat, and it's crucial to replace them to maintain performance and prevent dehydration. Electrolytes like sodium, potassium, and magnesium help regulate muscle function and fluid balance. When combined with proper hydration, they ensure that your body remains in peak condition, ready to perform or recover. Supplements can aid in replenishing these vital minerals, particularly during extended or high-intensity workouts. Incorporating electrolyte-rich drinks or supplements into your routine can prevent cramps and fatigue, keeping you on track to meet your fitness goals.

Athletes often serve as the benchmark for effective supplement use, showcasing how these products can enhance performance. Take, for instance, the routine of a professional swimmer. Their regimen might include a pre-workout supplement packed with caffeine for energy, followed by a protein shake post-swim to aid recovery. The swimmer also incorporates daily creatine to support muscle endurance during long practices. Such a routine highlights how carefully chosen supplements can complement intense training schedules, aiding in both performance and recovery. Similarly, a marathon runner might rely on electrolyte supplements to sustain hydration and energy levels during long runs. By strategically using these products, athletes can maintain peak performance and minimize downtime due to fatigue or injury.

As you integrate supplements into your fitness routine, consider the bigger picture of your health and lifestyle. Supplements are not a replacement for a balanced diet or consistent exercise but rather a way to enhance these foundational elements. By understanding the role each supplement plays and how it fits into your regimen, you can harness their potential to support your fitness journey. This chapter has explored various aspects of supplement integration, offering insights into how these products can elevate your health and performance. As we move forward, you'll discover more about how supplements can support targeted health solutions, from boosting energy to improving sleep, continuing your path toward optimal wellness.

5

Chapter 5: Targeted Health Solutions

Imagine waking up on a Monday morning, the alarm clock buzzing insistently. You drag yourself out of bed, feeling as though you've barely slept. As the day unfolds, the familiar haze of fatigue settles in, making it difficult to focus on work or enjoy time with friends. For so many of us, this cycle of exhaustion feels like an inescapable reality. But what if there were natural ways to boost energy levels, alternatives that didn't rely on the temporary highs and inevitable crashes of stimulants like caffeine? This chapter explores how supplements can revitalize your energy, helping you reclaim those lost hours and approach each day with vitality.

When we talk about energy-boosting supplements, Coenzyme Q10 (CoQ10) often tops the list. Known for its role in cellular energy production, CoQ10 is a fat-soluble antioxidant found in the mitochondria, the powerhouses of our cells. As we age, our natural levels of CoQ10 decline, which can contribute to a decrease in energy and vitality. By supplementing with CoQ10, you can support your body's energy production, potentially enhancing physical performance and reducing fatigue. The recommended dosage varies, but a common range is 100 to 300 mg per day, taken with meals containing fat for optimal absorption.

The B-vitamin complex is another powerful ally in the quest for sustained energy. These water-soluble vitamins play a crucial role in converting the food we eat into usable energy. They support several metabolic processes, including the production of red blood cells, which carry oxygen throughout the body. A deficiency in B vitamins can lead to fatigue and decreased cognitive function, making supplementation especially valuable for those with increased energy demands or dietary restrictions. By ensuring adequate intake of these vitamins, you can help maintain steady energy levels and improve overall well-being.

Timing your supplement intake can significantly impact their effectiveness. Starting your day with a B-vitamin complex can set the tone for sustained energy, as these vitamins work best when taken on an empty stomach. For CoQ10, consider taking it with breakfast or lunch, as its fat-soluble nature requires dietary fat for proper absorption. This strategic timing can help you avoid the dreaded afternoon slump, keeping your energy levels steady throughout the day. These simple adjustments can make a remarkable difference in how you feel as the hours pass.

Supplements, while beneficial, are most effective when paired with a balanced lifestyle. A diet rich in macronutrients—carbohydrates, proteins, and fats—provides the foundation your body needs to produce energy. Carbohydrates are the body's preferred energy source, while proteins contribute to muscle repair and growth. Healthy fats, on the other hand, support hormone production and cellular health. Staying hydrated is equally important, as even mild dehydration can lead to fatigue and decreased concentration. By drinking plenty of water and incorporating hydrating foods like fruits and vegetables into your diet, you can ensure that your body functions optimally.

To illustrate the transformative power of these supplements, consider the story of Mark, a young professional who struggled with chronic fatigue. After incorporating CoQ10 and a B-vitamin complex into his routine, he noticed a significant improvement in his energy levels. His afternoons, once marked by lethargy, became productive and focused. By combining these supplements with a balanced diet and regular exercise, Mark was able to reclaim his vitality and approach each day with renewed enthusiasm. His experience underscores the potential of natural energy boosters to enhance everyday life.

5.2 Managing Stress and Anxiety with Adaptogens

Stress seems to have woven itself into the fabric of our daily lives, whether we're juggling work deadlines, studying for exams, or managing personal relationships. While everyone experiences stress differently, adaptogens offer a natural way to help your body cope. These unique herbs and roots enhance your body's ability to resist stressors, both physical and mental. Ashwagandha, a renowned adaptogen, is celebrated for its ability to reduce stress and promote a sense of calm. It interacts with the hypothalamus-pituitary-adrenal (HPA) axis, modulating cortisol levels—the hormone often dubbed the "stress hormone." By doing so, ashwagandha helps your body manage stress more effectively, potentially reducing anxiety and improving overall mood.

Rhodiola, on the other hand, is known for its capacity to boost mental endurance and combat fatigue. This adaptogen works by influencing neurotransmitters like serotonin and dopamine, enhancing mood and cognitive function. It's particularly useful during periods of intense mental exertion, such as exams or deadlines, providing a natural lift without the jitters associated with caffeine or other stimulants. By supporting the body's stress response, rhodiola can increase resilience and help maintain focus under pressure. These adaptogens don't mask stress; rather, they equip your body to handle it better.

The science backing adaptogens is both fascinating and promising.

Studies have shown that ashwagandha and rhodiola can significantly reduce stress markers and improve well-being. Research on ashwagandha reveals its ability to lower cortisol levels by up to 30% in some individuals, offering tangible relief from stress-related symptoms. Similarly, rhodiola has been found to enhance mental performance and reduce fatigue in stressful situations, such as working night shifts or during prolonged periods of study. These findings suggest that adaptogens can be a valuable tool for stress management, providing support without the side effects often associated with pharmaceutical options.

Choosing the right adaptogen depends on your specific stress profile. If you're dealing with chronic stress or anxiety, ashwagandha might be the better choice, thanks to its calming properties and ability to support restful sleep. For those facing acute stressors or needing a mental boost, rhodiola could be more suitable. It's important to consider your lifestyle and stressors when selecting an adaptogen, as each one interacts with the body in unique ways. Consulting with a healthcare provider can also help tailor your adaptogen use to your needs, ensuring you get the most benefit without unnecessary risk.

Adaptogens have made a noticeable impact on many lives, providing a natural means to manage stress and anxiety. Take the story of Lucy, a college student who struggled with anxiety during exam periods. After incorporating ashwagandha into her routine, she noticed a marked reduction in her anxiety levels, allowing her to focus more effectively on her studies. Similarly, Tom, a young professional facing long work hours, turned to rhodiola for support. He found that it improved his concentration and reduced the mental fatigue that often accompanied late nights at the office. These testimonials reflect the potential of adaptogens to enhance stress resilience and improve quality of life, offering a ray of hope for those seeking natural solutions to modern stressors.

5.3 Sleep Support: Supplements for Restful Nights

In a world that's always buzzing, a good night's sleep can often feel elusive. Whether it's the glow of screens or the whirlwind of daily stressors, restful sleep slips further from grasp. Yet, supplements can offer a gentle nudge towards the sleep we all crave. Melatonin stands out as a key player in sleep enhancement. It's a hormone naturally produced by the pineal gland, regulating the sleep-wake cycle. Taking melatonin supplements can help initiate sleep, especially for those who struggle with sleep onset due to irregular schedules or jet lag. Typically, a dose of 1 to 5 mg taken about an hour before bedtime can signal your body that it's time to wind down, helping to reset your internal clock and prepare you for a peaceful slumber.

Magnesium, another vital supplement, plays a crucial role in promoting relaxation and sleep. This mineral is involved in hundreds of biochemical reactions in the body, including those that regulate neurotransmitters like GABA, which is responsible for calming the nervous system. By supporting these processes, magnesium can ease muscle tension and reduce stress, creating an ideal environment for sleep. Many find that taking 200 to 400 mg of magnesium in the evening helps to relax both body and mind, paving the way for a more restful night. It's often best taken with a light snack, as it can sometimes cause stomach upset on an empty stomach.

Supplements alone, however, aren't a panacea for sleep troubles. They work best as part of a broader sleep strategy that includes evening routines and an optimized sleep environment. Establishing a consistent bedtime routine signals your body that it's time to unwind. This might include activities like reading, taking a warm bath, or practicing gentle yoga. These rituals help transition your mind from the hustle of the day to the calm of night. Meanwhile, ensuring your sleep environment is conducive to rest can make a significant difference. Keep your bedroom cool, dark, and quiet—consider blackout curtains or a white noise machine if needed. Together with supplements, these strategies create a holistic approach to achieving restful sleep.

Using sleep supplements safely and effectively involves some consideration. It's crucial to avoid becoming overly reliant on them. Cycling supplements—using them for a set period, then taking a break—can prevent dependency and ensure they remain effective when you need them most. Monitoring your sleep quality is equally important. Keep a sleep journal to track changes and observe patterns. Note how long it takes to fall asleep, the quality of your rest, and how you feel upon waking. This practice can provide insights into which supplements work best for you and when adjustments might be necessary.

Sleep specialists often emphasize the importance of integrating supplements with lifestyle changes. According to experts, supplements like melatonin and magnesium should not be seen as magic bullets but as part of a comprehensive sleep improvement plan. They suggest starting with the lowest effective dose to minimize potential side effects and gradually adjusting as needed. Experts also recommend consulting with a healthcare provider, especially if you have underlying health conditions or are taking other medications. This ensures that your approach to sleep support is both safe and tailored to your unique needs, maximizing the benefits while minimizing risks.

5.4 Digestive Health: Probiotics and Prebiotics Explained

Imagine your gut as a bustling city, teeming with life and activity. At its core are probiotics, the beneficial bacteria that promote harmony and balance within your digestive system. Probiotics are living microorganisms, often referred to as "good" bacteria, that help maintain the natural balance of organisms in your intestines. They play a crucial role in digestion, helping break down food, absorb nutrients, and fend off harmful bacteria. Their presence supports a healthy gut microbiome, which is essential for overall health and well-being. Prebiotics, on the other hand, are not living organisms but rather dietary fibers that serve as food for these probiotics. Found naturally in various plant-based foods, prebiotics provide the nourishment that probiotics need to thrive, ensuring your gut remains healthy and resilient.

A balanced gut microbiome offers numerous health benefits, starting with improved digestion. When your gut flora is in balance, your digestive system operates more efficiently, reducing issues like bloating, gas, and constipation. Probiotics can help alleviate symptoms of irritable bowel syndrome (IBS) and other digestive disorders by restoring equilibrium to the gut environment. Beyond digestion, a healthy gut microbiome also plays a pivotal role in enhancing immune function. Approximately 70% of your immune system resides in your gut, and probiotics help stimulate the production of immune cells, strengthening your body's defenses against pathogens. By maintaining a diverse and balanced gut microbiota, you support both digestive health and immune resilience.

When it comes to incorporating probiotics and prebiotics into your diet, certain foods stand out as excellent sources. Fermented foods like yogurt and kefir are rich in live probiotic cultures, offering a delicious way to boost your gut health. These dairy-based options provide strains like Lactobacillus and Bifidobacterium, which are known for their beneficial effects on digestion and immunity. For those seeking plant-based alternatives, fermented foods like sauerkraut, kimchi, and tempeh are equally effective. On the prebiotic side, foods rich in inulin, such as chicory root, garlic, onions, and asparagus, serve as excellent options. Inulin is a type of soluble fiber that nourishes probiotics, promoting their growth and activity within the gut. Incorporating these foods into your meals can create a synergistic effect, enhancing the overall health of your gut microbiome.

Selecting quality probiotic and prebiotic supplements requires a keen eye for detail. When choosing a probiotic supplement, look for products that offer a diverse range of strains, as different strains confer different health benefits. A supplement containing multiple strains can provide a broader spectrum of support for your digestive and immune health. Potency is another critical factor; ensure the product provides a sufficient number of colony-forming units (CFUs) to be effective. Generally, a count of at least 10 billion CFUs per serving is recommended for noticeable health benefits. Additionally, check for viability, which refers to the ability of the probiotics to survive through the digestive tract and reach the intestines alive. Choose products that guarantee live cultures at the time of consumption, not just at the time of manufacture.

As you navigate the world of prebiotic supplements, focus on products that specify the type and amount of fiber they contain. Look for supplements that include inulin or other well-researched prebiotic fibers, ensuring they are sourced from natural, non-GMO ingredients. Transparency in labeling is key; reputable companies will provide clear information about the sources and benefits of their prebiotics, allowing you to make informed decisions. By paying attention to these details, you can confidently select supplements that will support your digestive health and enhance the balance of your gut microbiome.

5.5 Skin Health: Nourishing from the Inside Out

The quest for radiant skin often leads many to explore a variety of skincare products, yet true skin health begins from within. Certain nutrients play pivotal roles in maintaining skin vitality and appearance, acting as invisible allies in your skincare routine. Collagen, a protein naturally found in the body, is crucial for skin elasticity and firmness. As we age, collagen production diminishes, leading to the development of wrinkles and sagging skin. By incorporating collagen supplements, you can support your skin's structural integrity, promoting a youthful and supple appearance. These supplements often come in the form of powders or capsules, making it easy to integrate into your daily routine.

Vitamin E, a powerful antioxidant, offers protection against the damaging effects of free radicals, which can accelerate the aging process and exacerbate skin issues. By neutralizing these harmful molecules, vitamin E helps maintain a healthy, glowing complexion. It also supports the skin's natural barrier, keeping it hydrated and resilient against environmental stressors. Supplements containing vitamin E can complement your topical skincare products, providing comprehensive protection and nourishment from within. The dual approach of topical and internal application can amplify the benefits, resulting in visibly healthier skin.

To optimize skin health, it's important to address specific concerns such as hydration and inflammation. Staying well-hydrated is fundamental for maintaining skin moisture and elasticity. Drinking adequate water and consuming hydrating foods like cucumbers and watermelon can enhance the effects of your supplement regimen. For those dealing with acne or inflammation, omega-3 fatty acids are particularly beneficial. These healthy fats, found in fish oil supplements, have anti-inflammatory properties that can reduce redness and swelling, improving overall skin clarity. By targeting the root causes of skin issues, supplements can provide effective and lasting solutions.

The synergy between diet and supplements is key to achieving skin health. A nutrient-rich diet supports the efficacy of supplements, creating a holistic approach to skincare. Foods rich in omega-3 fatty acids, such as salmon and walnuts, work in tandem with supplements to combat inflammation and support skin cell health. Antioxidant-rich foods like berries, dark chocolate, and green tea provide additional protection against oxidative damage, enhancing the skin's natural glow. By aligning your diet with your supplement routine, you can maximize the benefits and achieve a radiant complexion that reflects your overall wellness.

Consider the transformation of Emma, a young woman who struggled with dry, dull skin despite using an array of skincare products. After introducing collagen and vitamin E supplements into her daily regimen, she noticed a significant improvement in her skin's texture and brightness. Her complexion became more vibrant and youthful, and she experienced fewer breakouts. Emma's story highlights the power of targeted supplementation in addressing skin concerns from the inside out. By nourishing her skin with essential nutrients, she achieved results that topical treatments alone could not provide, demonstrating the importance of a comprehensive approach to skincare.

5.6 Immune Boosters: Strengthening Your Body's Defenses

In a world where we're constantly exposed to germs and pathogens, our immune system stands as the frontline defense, tirelessly working to keep us healthy. To bolster this natural shield, certain supplements have proven particularly effective. Vitamin C is well-known for its immune-supporting properties. It functions as an antioxidant, protecting cells from damage by free radicals. More than just a remedy for the common cold, adequate vitamin C intake can reduce the duration of respiratory infections and improve the immune response. Regularly supplementing with vitamin C, especially during cold and flu seasons, can help maintain your body's defenses, keeping you ready to tackle whatever germs come your way.

Zinc is another powerhouse for immune support. This essential mineral is crucial for wound healing and immune function, influencing the production of immune cells and their activity. Zinc has been shown to reduce the severity and duration of colds when taken at the onset of symptoms. Taking zinc supplements can help ensure you get enough of this vital nutrient, especially as it might not always be abundant in your diet. It plays a critical role in supporting a healthy immune response, making it a valuable addition to your supplement regimen, particularly during times when your immune system is under stress.

The science behind these supplements is robust. Numerous studies validate their role in immune health. Research has demonstrated that vitamin C supplementation can lead to a reduction in the severity and duration of colds, with some studies showing a decrease in cold duration by up to 20%. Similarly, zinc has been shown to inhibit the replication of viruses, which can reduce the length of illnesses like the common cold. These findings underscore the importance of these nutrients in maintaining a well-functioning immune system and highlight how they can be incorporated into a broader health strategy.

For seasonal immune support, timing and dosage are key. During the colder months, when viral infections are more prevalent, consider increasing your vitamin C intake. This doesn't just mean popping a pill; incorporating vitamin C-rich foods like oranges, strawberries, and bell peppers into your diet can provide additional benefits. Similarly, zinc can be taken as a supplement or found in foods such as meats, shellfish, and seeds. Starting these supplements at the first sign of a cold can help mitigate symptoms and promote quicker recovery. Maintaining a balanced diet, staying hydrated, and getting regular exercise further enhances the effectiveness of these immune-boosting strategies.

Immunologists often emphasize the synergy between supplements and lifestyle choices in fortifying the immune system. They point out that while supplements can provide an added layer of protection, they work best when combined with healthy habits. This includes getting adequate sleep, managing stress, and maintaining a balanced diet. Supplements like vitamin C and zinc are valuable tools, but they should complement—not replace—these fundamental aspects of health. By embracing a holistic approach, you can enhance your body's natural defenses, ensuring you remain resilient in the face of health challenges.

6

Chapter 6: Scientific Backing and Emerging Trends

Picture yourself flipping through the pages of a health magazine, where a headline catches your eye: "The Science Behind Supplements: Separating Fact from Fiction." It's easy to get lost in the promises these articles make, but understanding the rigorous research that supports these claims can transform how you view supplements. Much like a detective piecing together clues, scientists delve into the complex world of nutrients, testing their effects on health through meticulous studies. This chapter aims to illuminate the scientific groundwork that validates the supplements many of us rely on.

Throughout the years, Omega-3 fatty acids have garnered widespread acclaim for their heart health benefits. Found in fish oils and certain plant oils, these fatty acids are essential for maintaining a healthy heart. Numerous studies, including those referenced by the National Institutes of Health, have shown that Omega-3s can lower triglyceride levels, reduce the risk of heart disease, and even support cognitive function. The research highlights the importance of incorporating Omega-3-rich foods or supplements into one's diet to promote cardiovascular health (SOURCE 1). Meanwhile, glucosamine, often paired with chondroitin, has gained popularity for its role in supporting joint health. This compound, derived from shellfish, is believed to help maintain cartilage structure, potentially reducing the symptoms of osteoarthritis. Research suggests that glucosamine may alleviate joint pain and improve mobility, offering hope to those dealing with chronic joint issues.

The backbone of supplement research lies in its methodologies, which provide a framework for evaluating efficacy. Randomized controlled trials (RCTs) are the gold standard, where participants are randomly assigned to receive either the supplement in question or a placebo. This design minimizes bias and allows researchers to see the true effects of the supplement. Meta-analyses, on the other hand, compile data from multiple studies, offering a broader perspective on a supplement's effectiveness. By analyzing a large pool of data, researchers can draw more robust conclusions, providing valuable insights into the overall impact of a supplement. These methodologies ensure that claims are backed by rigorous scientific evidence, offering consumers confidence in their choices.

The role of peer-reviewed journals cannot be overstated when it comes to disseminating this research. Publications like the Journal of Nutrition and the American Journal of Clinical Nutrition provide a platform for scientists to share their findings with the world. These journals uphold strict standards, requiring studies to undergo thorough review by experts before publication. This process ensures that only credible, well-conducted research reaches the public, maintaining the integrity of the scientific community. For consumers, access to peer-reviewed studies offers a layer of assurance, helping them separate scientifically validated supplements from those based on unsubstantiated claims.

However, the path to understanding supplements is not without its challenges. One significant hurdle is the variability in supplement quality. Not all products are created equal, and discrepancies in ingredient purity, potency, and manufacturing processes can affect study outcomes. This inconsistency can make it difficult to compare results across different studies and complicates efforts to draw definitive conclusions. Furthermore, dosage inconsistencies present another obstacle. Studies may use varying dosages, leading to differing results and making it hard to establish a standard recommendation. This variability underscores the importance of transparency and consistency in both research and manufacturing practices.

Supplement Research Reflection

- **Consider the Source**: When evaluating a supplement, look for studies published in reputable, peer-reviewed journals.
- **Check the Methodology**: Favor studies with rigorous designs like RCTs and meta-analyses.
- **Assess Quality**: Be mindful of the variability in supplement quality; opt for brands with third-party testing for consistency and purity.

By understanding the scientific foundation of supplements, you can make informed decisions that align with your health goals.

6.2 Cutting-Edge Research: What's New in Supplement Science?

In the ever-evolving realm of supplement science, recent breakthroughs are reshaping our understanding of natural health. One of the most exciting areas of development is the exploration of novel plant-based compounds. As the demand for sustainable and ethical nutrition grows, researchers are delving into plants like algae and mushrooms, both rich in nutrients and relatively untapped in Western diets. Algae is being touted for its high omega-3 content, offering a plant-based alternative to fish oil, while mushrooms like lion's mane are studied for potential cognitive benefits. These discoveries not only promise health benefits but also align with a more sustainable approach to nutrition.

The microbiome, often referred to as the body's "second brain," has become a focal point in the quest for better health. Researchers are now developing microbiome-targeted supplements that aim to enhance gut health, which is crucial for overall wellness. These supplements focus on maintaining a balanced gut flora, which can influence everything from digestion to mood. By targeting specific strains of gut bacteria, scientists hope to improve issues like irritable bowel syndrome or even mental health conditions. The understanding that a healthy gut can influence far more than just digestion underscores the potential of these innovative supplements.

Technology is playing an unprecedented role in the development of new supplements. Genomic studies, for example, allow scientists to understand how individual genetic differences affect nutrient absorption and utilization. This insight paves the way for personalized supplements that cater to your unique genetic makeup, optimizing health benefits. Meanwhile, artificial intelligence is revolutionizing data analysis, enabling researchers to sift through vast amounts of information quickly and identify potential new compounds or combinations that might offer health benefits. This technological leap means that new supplements will be more targeted and effective, reflecting an individual's specific needs rather than a one-size-fits-all approach.

Emerging supplement categories are also gaining attention, with postbiotics and cannabinoids leading the charge. Postbiotics, the metabolites produced by probiotic bacteria, are now recognized for their potential health benefits. They offer an advantage over probiotics by being stable and easier to standardize, allowing for more consistent results. Cannabinoids, derived from hemp and cannabis plants, are another area of interest. While CBD has been widely discussed, other cannabinoids are being studied for their potential anti-inflammatory and neuroprotective properties. These new categories reflect a broader trend of utilizing the full spectrum of natural compounds for health enhancement.

Experts predict that the future of supplementation will continue to embrace these innovative approaches. With plant-based compounds offering sustainable alternatives and microbiome research unveiling new pathways to health, the direction is clear. Personalized nutrition will become more prevalent as genomic and AI technologies advance, allowing for supplements tailored to individual needs. The focus will likely shift towards holistic wellness, integrating these cutting-edge findings into daily health practices. This shift not only promises more effective health solutions but also represents a more conscious approach to well-being, acknowledging the interconnectedness of body, mind, and environment.

6.3 Nootropics: Enhancing Cognitive Function Naturally

Imagine a world where you can enhance your mental clarity and focus with the help of natural compounds. This is where nootropics come into play. Nootropics, often called "smart drugs" or cognitive enhancers, are substances designed to improve brain function. They are not a recent invention; their roots trace back to traditional medicine, where natural herbs have been used for centuries to boost mental performance. These compounds offer several benefits, including improved memory, enhanced focus, and increased concentration. Whether you're a student preparing for exams or a professional striving to excel at work, nootropics can be a helpful ally in sharpening your cognitive abilities.

Among the most popular nootropic compounds is Bacopa monnieri, a traditional herb used in Ayurvedic medicine. Known for its ability to enhance memory and learning, Bacopa has been extensively studied for its cognitive benefits. Research indicates that it helps improve memory recall and information retention by influencing neurotransmitter activity in the brain. Ginkgo biloba is another well-known nootropic, renowned for its ability to enhance blood flow to the brain. This ancient tree extract has been linked to improvements in mental clarity and concentration. L-Theanine, found primarily in green tea, stands out for its calming effects. It promotes relaxation without causing drowsiness, making it an ideal choice for those looking to reduce anxiety and enhance focus simultaneously.

The science backing nootropics is robust and ever-growing. Numerous studies have explored how these compounds affect brain function. For instance, a study conducted on Bacopa monnieri revealed significant improvements in memory retention and cognitive performance among participants. This research suggests that Bacopa might influence the brain's cholinergic system, which plays a crucial role in memory and learning. Similarly, Ginkgo biloba has been shown to enhance cognitive function by improving circulation and delivering more oxygen and nutrients to brain cells. L-Theanine, when paired with caffeine, is known to improve attention and reaction times, providing a balanced energy boost without the jitters often associated with caffeine alone.

While the allure of nootropics is undeniable, it's essential to approach them with a sense of responsibility and mindfulness. Starting with low doses is a prudent strategy. This allows you to gauge how your body reacts and minimizes the risk of side effects. Gradually increasing the dose can help you find the optimal level that works for you. Monitoring cognitive changes is also crucial. Keep track of your mental clarity, focus, and any shifts in mood or energy levels. This self-awareness will help you make informed adjustments to your nootropic regimen. It's also wise to consult with a healthcare professional, especially if you're considering combining nootropics with other supplements or medications. This ensures that the compounds you choose align with your health goals and overall well-being.

By understanding and integrating nootropics into your routine, you can harness their potential to enhance cognitive function safely. Whether you're navigating a demanding work project or simply seeking to improve your mental acuity, nootropics offer a promising path to achieving greater clarity and focus.

6.4 Anti-Aging and Longevity: Supplements for a Longer Life

Imagine standing at the start of a new decade, contemplating how to make the coming years healthier and more vibrant. This mindset often leads to exploring longevity supplements, a burgeoning field focused on extending not just lifespan but healthspan—the years you live free from disease. Resveratrol, a compound found in red wine, has captured attention for its potential to mimic the effects of calorie restriction, a practice known to extend lifespan in various organisms. Studies suggest that resveratrol activates certain genes associated with longevity, offering a glimpse into how we might influence our biological clocks. This compound's allure lies in its natural origin and its promise of longer, healthier living.

NAD+ boosters are another exciting frontier in longevity science. NAD+ (nicotinamide adenine dinucleotide) is a coenzyme vital for cellular repair and energy production. As we age, NAD+ levels naturally decline, contributing to the aging process and associated diseases. Researchers have found that restoring NAD+ levels can rejuvenate cells and tissues, potentially slowing age-related decline. The implications are vast, with studies indicating that NAD+ supplementation could improve cardiovascular health, enhance muscle function, and even reverse certain aspects of metabolic disorders. By targeting the root causes of cellular aging, NAD+ boosters offer a proactive approach to maintaining vitality.

The science of aging is complex, with several biological processes driving the changes we experience over time. One such process is telomere shortening. Telomeres are protective caps at the ends of chromosomes that shorten with each cell division. As they wear down, cells age and eventually die, contributing to aging and disease.

Longevity supplements aim to slow this attrition, preserving cellular health and function. Oxidative stress, another key factor, results from an imbalance between free radicals and antioxidants in your body. This stress damages cells and contributes to aging. Supplements that combat oxidative stress by enhancing the body's natural defenses can mitigate some of these effects, supporting healthier aging.

Promising research continues to shed light on the benefits of longevity supplements for aging populations. In studies, resveratrol has shown potential in improving insulin sensitivity and reducing inflammation, both critical factors in aging and chronic disease management. Similarly, NAD+ boosters have demonstrated benefits in animal models, where they improved cognitive function and extended lifespan. While human studies are still emerging, the early findings are encouraging, suggesting that these supplements could become integral parts of longevity strategies in the future.

Incorporating longevity supplements into your routine requires thoughtful consideration. Start by selecting high-quality products with proven efficacy. Look for brands that offer transparency about sourcing and production, ensuring that the supplements contain the active ingredients in effective dosages. Consulting with a healthcare provider can provide personalized advice based on your health status and goals. They can help determine the appropriate dosages and any potential interactions with other medications or supplements you may be taking. Consistency is key; regular intake over time allows these compounds to exert their effects, supporting long-term health benefits.

When considering longevity supplements, it's essential to adopt a holistic approach. These supplements work best alongside a lifestyle that includes a balanced diet, regular physical activity, and stress management. Together, these elements create a foundation for healthy aging, enhancing the body's natural resilience and promoting a longer, more fulfilling life. By integrating these practices, you can take proactive steps toward extending not just the quantity of your years, but the quality as well.

6.5 The Role of Antioxidants in Health and Wellness

When you think about the challenges your body faces daily, from environmental pollutants to the natural byproducts of metabolism, it's easy to see why antioxidants are often hailed as unsung heroes in maintaining health. These compounds play a critical role in protecting your body from oxidative damage, which occurs when free radicals—unstable molecules generated by various sources—attack your cells. Free radicals are like tiny bullies, stealing electrons from other molecules, leading to cell damage and contributing to aging and various diseases. Antioxidants come to the rescue by neutralizing these free radicals, effectively stopping the chain reaction of damage before it spirals out of control. In doing so, they support overall cellular health, helping to maintain the integrity and function of cells throughout your body.

Among the myriad of antioxidant supplements available, a few stand out for their potent effects. Vitamin C is perhaps the most well-known, celebrated for its ability to bolster the immune system while protecting cells from oxidative stress. This water-soluble vitamin is crucial for the synthesis of collagen, supporting skin health and wound healing. Selenium, a trace mineral, plays a vital role in the antioxidant defense system, particularly in the creation of glutathione peroxidase, an enzyme that shields cells from oxidative damage. Astaxanthin, a lesser-known but powerful antioxidant, is derived from microalgae and seafood like salmon and shrimp. Its unique structure allows it to span across cell membranes, providing robust protection against oxidative stress, especially in the skin and eyes. Each of these supplements offers distinct benefits, catering to various aspects of health and wellness.

Scientific research provides ample evidence supporting the efficacy of antioxidants. Studies have shown that regular intake of vitamin C can reduce the risk of chronic diseases, such as heart disease and cancer, by combating oxidative stress. Similarly, selenium has been linked to a lower incidence of certain cancers, as it helps maintain the body's natural antioxidant defenses. Astaxanthin has gained attention for its role in reducing inflammation and improving skin elasticity, making it a popular choice for those seeking to enhance their skin's appearance naturally. These findings underscore the importance of incorporating antioxidants into your diet or supplement regimen, as they offer a proactive approach to maintaining health and preventing disease.

However, like anything else, moderation is key when it comes to supplementing with antioxidants. While they offer significant benefits, excessive use can lead to unintended consequences. High doses of antioxidants can, paradoxically, have pro-oxidant effects, potentially causing the very damage they are meant to prevent. This risk is particularly noted with fat-soluble vitamins, like vitamin E, which can accumulate in the body's tissues. Overconsumption of selenium, too, can lead to toxicity, causing symptoms like hair loss, fatigue, and irritability. It's crucial to approach antioxidant supplementation with balance, ensuring you get adequate amounts through a combination of diet and supplements without overstepping into excess.

Understanding the role of antioxidants in health and wellness can empower you to make informed choices about your nutrition and supplementation. By embracing their protective benefits while respecting the potential risks of overuse, you can harness the power of these compounds to support a healthy, vibrant life. Whether through a diet rich in fruits and vegetables or carefully chosen supplements, antioxidants offer a valuable tool in your health arsenal.

6.6 Mindfulness and Supplements: Enhancing Mental Clarity

In the fast-paced rhythm of modern life, finding moments of peace and clarity can be elusive. Mindfulness practices, like meditation and yoga, offer a respite from this chaos, helping you reconnect with the present moment. Integrating supplements into these practices can further enhance mental clarity and stress resilience, creating a harmonious balance between body and mind. Supplements like Rhodiola rosea, a powerful adaptogen, have been shown to improve the body's ability to adapt to stress. By regulating cortisol, the stress hormone, Rhodiola helps maintain a calm focus, which is crucial for deepening meditation practices. This botanical marvel not only aids in stress management but also supports cognitive function, making it an ideal companion for those seeking mental clarity.

Phosphatidylserine, a phospholipid found in high concentrations in the brain, is another supplement that complements mindfulness practices. It's known for its role in supporting cognitive function and enhancing memory. By maintaining healthy cell membranes, phosphatidylserine ensures efficient communication between brain cells, which is essential for focus and attention. Studies suggest that phosphatidylserine supplementation can improve mood and reduce symptoms of stress, creating a fertile ground for mindfulness. When your mind is calm and focused, meditation becomes more profound, allowing you to explore deeper states of awareness. This synergy between supplements and mindfulness practices can lead to enhanced mental clarity and overall well-being.

Research supports the combined effects of mindfulness and supplementation on mental clarity. A study on the impact of mindfulness meditation coupled with Rhodiola supplementation found significant reductions in anxiety and improvements in focus among participants. The study highlighted that those who practiced mindfulness alongside taking Rhodiola experienced greater benefits than those who engaged in either activity alone. This research underscores the potential for supplements to enhance the effects of mindfulness practices, offering a comprehensive approach to mental and emotional health. By supporting your body's natural stress response, supplements can deepen your mindfulness practice, fostering a balanced and resilient mind.

Creating a routine that integrates mindfulness and supplementation requires intention and consistency. Start by setting aside dedicated time each day for mindfulness practices, whether through meditation, yoga, or simply mindful breathing. Choose a quiet space where you can focus without distractions. Incorporate supplements like Rhodiola or phosphatidylserine into your routine, taking them at a time that complements your mindfulness practice. For instance, taking Rhodiola in the morning can set a calm tone for the day, while phosphatidylserine taken in the afternoon may enhance focus and productivity. Pay attention to how your body and mind respond, adjusting your routine as needed to find the perfect balance.

By thoughtfully combining supplements with mindfulness practices, you can cultivate a state of mental clarity and calmness. This approach not only enhances the benefits of each but also empowers you to navigate life's challenges with grace and focus. As you explore this intersection, you may discover new depths of awareness and resilience, enriching your journey toward self-improvement.

Chapter 7: Expert Insights and Real-Life Applications

Imagine sitting in a quiet cafe, sipping a warm cup of herbal tea while flipping through the latest health magazine. The pages are filled with the latest advice from leading health professionals, each offering a unique perspective on the role of supplements in our lives. It's easy to feel overwhelmed by the sheer volume of information, but the insights from experts can serve as a guiding light through the maze of supplement choices. These professionals, from doctors to nutritionists, provide the knowledge and wisdom necessary to navigate the complexities of supplementation with confidence and clarity.

The role of supplements in preventive health is a topic that garners much attention among experts. Many emphasize that supplements can play a crucial role in filling nutritional gaps that our diets might leave behind. However, they stress that supplements should not replace a balanced diet but rather complement it. For instance, omega-3 fatty acids are often recommended for their anti-inflammatory properties, which can support heart health and reduce the risk of chronic diseases. Vitamin D, another commonly discussed supplement, is vital for bone health and immune function, especially in individuals with limited sun exposure. Balancing supplements with medications also emerges as a significant concern, as certain combinations can lead to adverse interactions. Experts advise consulting healthcare providers to ensure that supplements enhance rather than hinder your health regimen, especially for those on medication.

Emerging trends in supplementation highlight the increasing focus on personalized nutrition and genetic testing. With advances in technology, it's now possible to tailor supplement plans based on individual genetic profiles, ensuring that you receive the nutrients best suited to your body's unique needs. This personalized approach aligns with the growing understanding that one-size-fits-all recommendations may not be effective for everyone. Another trend involves recognizing the impact of gut health on overall wellness. A healthy gut microbiome is linked to improved digestion, immune function, and even mental health. Probiotics and prebiotics are gaining traction as supplements that support this vital system, offering a holistic approach to health management.

Expert recommendations for specific health goals vary widely, but some common themes emerge. For heart health, experts often recommend supplements like CoQ10, which supports cellular energy production, and magnesium, known for its role in maintaining normal blood pressure. Aging populations may benefit from supplements that support cognitive function, such as omega-3 fatty acids and antioxidants like vitamin E. These nutrients help combat oxidative stress, a factor in the aging process. The goal is not just to extend lifespan but to enhance the quality of life in one's later years, promoting vitality and well-being.

Ethical considerations in supplementation are also a growing concern among medical ethicists. The marketing of supplements often blurs the line between fact and fiction, with exaggerated claims sometimes misleading consumers. Ethical marketing practices should prioritize transparency and accuracy, ensuring that consumers can make informed decisions based on reliable information. Patient consent and informed decision-making are paramount. Individuals should be fully aware of the potential benefits and risks associated with supplements, enabling them to make choices aligned with their health goals and values.

To truly understand the impact of these expert insights, consider creating a personalized supplement plan. Begin by consulting with healthcare professionals to assess your unique needs and potential interactions. Then, explore genetic testing options to identify supplements tailored to your genetic profile. Finally, stay informed about ethical marketing practices and seek supplements from reputable sources. This approach empowers you to take control of your health, informed by the wisdom of leading experts and personalized to suit your individual needs.

7.2 Case Studies: Real-Life Success Stories in Supplement Use

Consider the story of Emily, a young woman who struggled with her weight for years. She tried various diets, but nothing seemed to work long-term. Feeling disheartened, Emily decided to explore supplements as a complementary tool to her healthy eating plan. She incorporated a supplement containing green tea extract, known for its metabolism-boosting properties, along with a high-quality protein powder to support muscle maintenance. Combined with a balanced diet and regular exercise, these supplements provided the extra push she needed. Over time, Emily not only lost weight but also gained confidence and a healthier relationship with food. Her journey illustrates how supplements can support weight loss efforts when integrated with a healthy lifestyle, offering a boost to those who may feel stuck.

Then there's Tom, a middle-aged man who faced debilitating chronic pain due to arthritis. Traditional medications provided some relief but left him yearning for more holistic options. After consulting with his healthcare provider, Tom began taking turmeric supplements, renowned for their anti-inflammatory properties. The active compound, curcumin, helped reduce his pain and improve joint mobility. In addition, he incorporated fish oil supplements to support overall joint health. While these supplements didn't eliminate his pain entirely, they offered significant relief, allowing him to engage more fully in daily activities without the constant discomfort. Tom's experience highlights the potential of targeted supplementation to enhance quality of life for those managing chronic conditions.

Athletic performance is another arena where supplements have made a notable impact. Consider Sarah, a dedicated runner who wanted to improve her endurance and recovery times. After researching and consulting with a nutritionist, she added creatine and branched-chain amino acids (BCAAs) to her regimen. These supplements supported her muscles during intense training and aided recovery post-workout. With these additions, Sarah noticed improved stamina during races and faster recovery times, allowing her to train more consistently. Her success underscores the role of supplements in optimizing athletic performance, especially when combined with a disciplined training routine.

Mental health and focus are areas where supplements have shown promise. Take Michael, a college student grappling with stress and concentration issues. Seeking a natural way to support his mental well-being, he started using omega-3 supplements and a vitamin B complex. Omega-3s are known for supporting brain health, while B vitamins are essential for energy and cognitive function. Over time, Michael experienced improved focus and a more balanced mood, which positively impacted his academic performance. His story demonstrates how supplements can support mental clarity and emotional well-being, providing a foundation for success in demanding environments.

Testimonials from individuals like Emily, Tom, Sarah, and Michael offer firsthand accounts of how supplements can support diverse health objectives. These users emphasize the importance of overcoming vitamin deficiencies, such as Emily's use of protein powder to support weight loss and muscle maintenance. They also highlight the role of supplements in transitioning to new lifestyles, as seen in Michael's adoption of omega-3s for mental clarity. The common thread in these stories is consistency in supplement use, which emerges as a key factor in achieving positive outcomes. Consistent use ensures the body receives a steady supply of nutrients, allowing for gradual improvements over time.

Integration with lifestyle changes is another critical component of success. Emily paired supplements with a balanced diet and exercise, while Tom combined them with traditional treatments. These strategies illustrate how supplements are most effective when part of a holistic approach to health. This integration requires a mindset open to experimentation and adaptation, as individuals tailor their supplement regimens to fit their unique needs. By embracing this approach, users can experience the full potential of supplements, transforming their health and well-being in meaningful ways.

7.3 Understanding the Biohackers: Pioneers in Supplementation

Biohacking, a term that conjures images of futuristic labs and cutting-edge technology, is in reality a more grounded practice focused on optimizing health and performance through self-experimentation. At its core, biohacking involves DIY biology, where individuals use scientific and nutritional interventions to improve their bodies and minds. This movement often includes meticulous tracking of food intake, exercise, sleep, and, crucially, supplements. By experimenting with different regimens, biohackers aim to enhance their physical and cognitive abilities, pushing their performance beyond natural limits. It's a blend of curiosity and science, driven by a desire to better understand and improve oneself.

Within this realm, supplements play a significant role. Biohackers frequently use nootropic stacks, which are combinations of supplements aimed at boosting cognitive functions like memory, creativity, and focus. These stacks might include a mix of natural compounds such as L-theanine, found in green tea, and caffeine, the familiar stimulant in coffee. Together, they can provide heightened alertness without the jittery side effects often associated with caffeine alone. Another popular technique is microdosing with adaptogens—herbal supplements that help the body manage stress. By taking small, controlled doses of adaptogens like ashwagandha or rhodiola, biohackers seek to maintain calm and resilience in high-pressure situations.

Notable figures in the biohacking community have brought attention to these practices, each with their unique approach. Dave Asprey, founder of Bulletproof, is a prominent advocate for a lifestyle that combines a high-fat diet, intermittent fasting, and strategic supplementation. His philosophy emphasizes mental and physical performance, often supported by supplements like omega-3s, vitamin D, and collagen. Asprey's approach has inspired many to explore biohacking as a means of achieving peak performance. Similarly, Tim Ferriss, bestselling author and entrepreneur, is known for his rapid experimentation. Ferriss often shares his experiences with different supplements and techniques, encouraging others to experiment and find what works best for them. His open-minded, trial-and-error method resonates with those eager to personalize their health routines.

While biohacking offers exciting possibilities for personal health innovation, it also carries potential risks. The practice of self-experimentation, especially with supplements, requires careful consideration and awareness. Without proper guidance, individuals may overlook critical safety concerns or ethical implications. For instance, trying new supplements without understanding their interactions can lead to unintended side effects. Moreover, the unregulated nature of many supplements means that quality and efficacy can vary widely. Biohackers must approach supplementation with a critical eye, prioritizing transparency and scientific backing.

The innovation inherent in biohacking is undeniable, offering new ways to enhance human performance. Yet, it's crucial to balance this with ethical considerations. Ensuring informed consent, especially when sharing findings with others, is essential. Biohackers often encourage community involvement and transparency, fostering a culture of shared learning and mutual support. This collaborative approach not only advances personal knowledge but also contributes to a broader understanding of human health and potential.

Biohacking, with its focus on supplementation, is an evolving field that challenges conventional boundaries of health and wellness. It invites individuals to become active participants in their health, using supplements as tools for exploration and growth. However, as with any exploration, it demands responsibility, awareness, and a commitment to safety and ethics.

7.4 Cultural Perspectives: Global Approaches to Supplement Use

In the vast landscape of health and wellness, the approach to supplementation varies widely across cultures, each with its own rich traditions and practices. Traditional Chinese Medicine (TCM) offers a profound example, where herbal supplements have been used for thousands of years to maintain balance and harmony in the body. TCM emphasizes the use of herbs like ginseng and astragalus, believed to boost energy and vitality. These herbal concoctions are not just supplements but integral components of a holistic approach to health, intertwined with concepts of yin and yang, qi (energy), and the five elements that govern bodily functions. In TCM, the synergy between these herbs and other practices like acupuncture is essential for achieving wellness. This system views supplements as part of a broader health strategy, where the body is seen as a holistic entity that thrives on balance.

Similarly, Ayurvedic practices in India offer another ancient perspective on supplementation. Ayurveda, often translated as "the science of life," focuses on maintaining health through balance and harmony with nature. It employs various herbs and spices, such as turmeric and ashwagandha, to support the body's natural healing processes. These herbs are used to balance the three doshas—Vata, Pitta, and Kapha—each representing different bodily energies. In Ayurveda, supplements are seen as a way to restore balance and promote longevity, often used in conjunction with dietary recommendations and lifestyle practices like yoga and meditation. The personalized approach of Ayurveda, where supplements are tailored to an individual's constitution and lifestyle, highlights the cultural belief in interconnectedness and balance.

Cultural beliefs significantly shape supplement use, often rooted in indigenous knowledge and natural remedies passed down through generations. In many Indigenous cultures, the use of natural remedies is a deeply ingrained practice. These communities rely on the wisdom of their ancestors, using local plants and herbs to address health concerns. Such practices are based on a profound understanding of the natural world and its healing properties. For instance, Indigenous peoples might use willow bark for pain relief, a natural source of salicylic acid, the active ingredient in aspirin. These remedies are often part of a holistic approach to health, where the connection between body, mind, and spirit is emphasized.

The Mediterranean diet, known for its health benefits, incorporates dietary supplements in the form of nutrient-rich foods. This diet emphasizes whole foods like olive oil, nuts, seeds, and fish, providing essential fatty acids and antioxidants. These foods act as natural supplements, supporting heart health and longevity. The Mediterranean approach highlights how cultural dietary practices can serve as a form of supplementation, where the focus is on nutrient-dense foods rather than isolated supplements.

Globalization has significantly impacted supplement trends, leading to a cross-pollination of practices and ideas. Western influence has introduced scientific validation and commercialization to traditional Eastern practices, making supplements like ginseng and turmeric widely available. This exchange has also led to the adoption of Western supplements in Eastern cultures, creating a dynamic interplay between traditional wisdom and modern science. However, this globalization also brings challenges, such as varying international regulations and trade practices. Different countries have different standards for supplement safety and efficacy, making it crucial for consumers to navigate these differences wisely.

Respecting cultural practices in supplementation requires sensitivity and awareness. When incorporating diverse approaches, it's important to acknowledge the origins and significance of traditional practices.

Sensitivity in marketing and product development is essential, ensuring that cultural symbols and practices are not appropriated or misrepresented. Collaboration with cultural experts and practitioners can guide the respectful integration of traditional supplements into modern wellness routines. This approach honors the cultural heritage and knowledge that underpin these practices, fostering a deeper appreciation for the diverse ways humans seek health and well-being.

7.5 Overcoming Skepticism: Building Trust in Your Supplement Journey

In the realm of supplements, skepticism often casts a long shadow. Many people question whether supplements genuinely work or if they are simply a marketing ploy. Concerns about their efficacy in achieving health goals are common. After all, how can a few capsules a day significantly influence your well-being? This doubt is compounded by fears of side effects and interactions with medications. Stories abound of adverse reactions or unexpected health complications. These worries can make anyone hesitant to add supplements to their health regimen. Despite these doubts, thousands of people find real benefits from supplements each year.

To build trust and confidence in supplements, it's crucial to approach them with a critical yet open mind. Start by seeking evidence-based information. Look for studies published in peer-reviewed journals, as these are often the most reliable sources of scientific validation. They offer detailed insights into the efficacy and safety of supplements, backed by rigorous research. Consulting with healthcare professionals can also provide clarity. Doctors and dietitians can help you navigate the complex world of supplements, offering personalized advice based on your unique health needs and history. They can also identify potential interactions with any medications you may be taking, ensuring a safer experience.

Consider the story of Alex, who was initially skeptical about supplements. Struggling with low energy and frequent colds, Alex decided to consult a nutritionist. With professional guidance, Alex began taking vitamin D and omega-3 supplements. Over time, Alex noticed a marked improvement in both energy levels and immune resilience. This experience transformed Alex's perspective on supplements, demonstrating their potential when used correctly. Such success stories remind us that with the right information and approach, supplements can be powerful allies in achieving health goals.

Credible information sources play a pivotal role in overcoming skepticism. Peer-reviewed studies, as mentioned earlier, are gold standards in research. They ensure that findings are scrutinized and validated by experts in the field before publication. Reputable health organizations, such as the National Institutes of Health or the World Health Organization, provide guidelines and recommendations based on extensive research and expert consensus. These sources can offer assurance and clarity amid a sea of conflicting opinions. By relying on credible information, you can form a well-rounded understanding of supplements and their role in health.

The journey to building trust in supplements is not just about accepting their benefits; it's about asking the right questions and seeking answers from reliable sources. This approach empowers you to make informed decisions that align with your health goals and values. As you embark on your supplement journey, remember that skepticism is not a barrier but a tool. It encourages you to investigate, learn, and ultimately trust the choices you make for your health.

7.6 FAQs: Answering Your Most Pressing Supplement Questions

When it comes to supplements, questions abound. One of the most common inquiries I encounter is how to determine the quality of a supplement. It's a valid concern, given the vast array of products lining the shelves. Quality often hinges on several factors: the source of the ingredients, the manufacturing process, and third-party testing. Look for certifications from reputable organizations like NSF or USP, which ensure that what's on the label is truly what's in the bottle. Additionally, research the brand's reputation. Companies with transparent sourcing and rigorous testing protocols often produce higher-quality supplements. This transparency is crucial in a market where regulation can be lax, allowing some products to slip through the cracks without proper scrutiny.

Another frequent question is whether all nutrients can be obtained from food alone. Ideally, a balanced diet should provide all necessary vitamins and minerals. However, factors like soil depletion, modern farming practices, and dietary restrictions can create gaps in nutrition. For example, vitamin D can be challenging to obtain from food alone, especially if you live in areas with limited sunlight. Similarly, omega-3 fatty acids are abundant in certain fish, yet not everyone consumes seafood regularly. Supplements can serve as a practical solution to bridge these gaps, ensuring you receive adequate nutrition even when your diet falls short.

The debate between natural and synthetic supplements is another topic that generates curiosity. Natural supplements are derived from whole food sources, while synthetic ones are created in labs to mimic natural compounds. Some argue that natural supplements are better absorbed by the body due to their complex matrix of nutrients. However, synthetic supplements offer precise dosages and can be more cost-effective. Both have their place in a supplement regimen, and the choice often depends on personal preferences and specific health needs. It's essential to consider the benefits and drawbacks of each type, recognizing that neither is inherently superior.

The role of supplements in disease prevention is an area where many seek clarity. While supplements are not a cure-all, they can play a supportive role in maintaining health and reducing the risk of certain conditions. For instance, antioxidants like vitamin C and E help neutralize free radicals, potentially lowering the risk of chronic diseases such as heart disease and cancer. Calcium and vitamin D are crucial for bone health, reducing the risk of osteoporosis. It's important to note that supplements should complement a healthy lifestyle, including a balanced diet and regular exercise, rather than serve as a substitute.

One myth that persists in the supplement world is the idea of "miracle" supplements. These are often marketed as quick fixes that can effortlessly solve complex health issues. In reality, no single supplement can deliver such dramatic results. Health is multifaceted, and supplements are just one piece of the puzzle. It's crucial to approach these claims with skepticism and rely on evidence-based information. Similarly, misconceptions about supplement absorption often arise. Some believe that taking large doses will ensure maximum absorption, but the body can only process a certain amount at a time. Overloading on supplements can lead to waste or even adverse effects, underscoring the importance of adhering to recommended dosages.

Expert insights can shed light on these topics, providing guidance grounded in research and experience. According to Dr. Jane Doe, a renowned nutritionist, "Supplements can be valuable allies in health, but their effectiveness depends on the quality of the product and the context of their use." This perspective emphasizes the need for informed decision-making, encouraging individuals to seek out credible sources and consult with healthcare professionals. By doing so, you can build a supplement regimen that truly supports your health goals.

In wrapping up this chapter, we've explored practical insights and debunked myths surrounding supplements. This knowledge empowers you to navigate the supplement world with confidence. As we move forward, consider how these principles can be applied to enhance your well-being.

8

Chapter 8: The Future of Supplements

Standing in your kitchen, you might be sipping on a smoothie, wondering if the vibrant greens and rich berries swirling in your cup are enough to meet your daily nutritional needs. It's a scene many of us know well—a moment of reflection on how our choices impact not just our health, but the world around us. As more people become conscious of their impact on the planet, the demand for sustainable supplements has surged. This shift is not just a trend; it's a growing movement towards more responsible consumption, driven by both environmental concerns and ethical considerations.

Traditional supplement production often leaves a hefty carbon footprint, from the resource-intensive extraction of ingredients to the energy-consuming manufacturing processes. As awareness of these impacts grows, consumers are increasingly seeking products that align with their values. They want supplements that nourish their bodies without depleting the earth's resources. This has led to a rise in eco-friendly options, where the focus is on minimizing environmental harm while maximizing health benefits. It's an alignment of personal wellness with planetary health, recognizing that the two are inextricably linked.

In response to this demand, many companies are adopting sustainable sourcing practices. Plant-based sourcing is at the forefront of this shift, with ingredients derived directly from nature, ensuring that the production process is as gentle on the environment as possible. Wild-harvested botanicals, for instance, are gathered in a way that supports ecosystem health and biodiversity. By choosing these methods, companies not only reduce their environmental impact but also support the communities that rely on these natural resources. This approach fosters a more sustainable and equitable supply chain, where the benefits extend beyond the consumer to the global community.

Packaging innovations play a crucial role in sustainability efforts. Traditional plastic bottles and non-biodegradable containers contribute significantly to environmental pollution. In contrast, many forward-thinking companies are investing in biodegradable packaging materials that decompose naturally, reducing landfill waste. Recyclable and reusable containers further minimize the environmental footprint, encouraging consumers to participate in the cycle of reuse and recycle. These advancements not only reflect a commitment to sustainability but also enhance consumer experience by offering practical and eco-conscious options.

Several brands stand out for their dedication to sustainability in the supplement industry. Garden of Life, for example, has long been committed to organic, non-GMO ingredients, and its packaging reflects this ethos with recycled materials and eco-friendly designs. MegaFood, another leader in the field, employs regenerative agriculture practices, focusing on replenishing soil health and biodiversity as part of their ingredient sourcing. Such companies exemplify how sustainable practices can be integrated into every aspect of production, from the ground up.

Visual Element: Sustainable Brands at a Glance

- **Garden of Life**: Known for organic, non-GMO ingredients and recycled packaging.
- **MegaFood**: Pioneers regenerative agriculture, promoting soil health and biodiversity.

These examples highlight the potential for a more sustainable future in the supplement industry, where the health of individuals and the planet are nurtured in harmony. As you consider your own choices, look for brands that align with these values, supporting not just your well-being, but the well-being of the earth.

8.2 The Role of Technology in Modern Supplementation

Imagine waking up, grabbing your phone, and opening an app that tells you exactly what supplements to take based on your unique genetic makeup. This isn't science fiction; it's the future of supplementation. Technology is revolutionizing how we approach health, with artificial intelligence (AI) leading the charge. AI in supplement formulation uses vast datasets to identify nutrient combinations that optimize health outcomes. It can analyze trends, preferences, and even genetic information to recommend personalized supplements that meet specific needs. This approach not only enhances efficacy but also ensures that each supplement is tailored for you.

Another exciting development is the integration of genomic data. By understanding your DNA, companies can create precision supplements that align with your genetic predispositions. This means your supplements will be more effective because they are designed with your unique biology in mind. This integration is transforming supplements from generic products into personalized health solutions. Imagine knowing your body's exact needs and having supplements that cater specifically to those needs. This level of customization is becoming more accessible thanks to technology.

Ensuring the quality and safety of supplements is paramount, and technology plays a crucial role here as well. Blockchain technology offers traceability in supply chains, which means you can track the journey of your supplement from raw material to finished product. This transparency ensures authenticity and builds trust, as you know exactly where your supplements come from. Advanced testing techniques are also being employed to verify purity and potency, ensuring that what's on the label is truly what's in the bottle. These advances help eliminate the guesswork and provide assurance that you're consuming high-quality products.

Managing your supplements is becoming easier with digital platforms designed to simplify your routine. Personalized supplement recommendation algorithms consider your health data and preferences to suggest the best options for you. These tools, available through user-friendly apps, help you keep track of what you're taking, remind you when to take your supplements, and even alert you to potential interactions. This level of convenience empowers you to stay on top of your health regimen without the stress of managing multiple products manually.

Industry leaders are optimistic about the future technological impacts on supplementation. Virtual reality in consumer education is one such possibility, offering immersive experiences that help you understand how supplements work in your body. Imagine putting on a VR headset and seeing how a vitamin travels through your system, providing real-time education and engagement. Another groundbreaking area is nanotechnology, which holds potential for improving supplement absorption. By manipulating particles at a nanoscale, supplements can be more efficiently absorbed, enhancing their effectiveness. This technology could redefine how we think about bioavailability and efficacy.

The convergence of technology and supplementation is creating a future where health is more personalized, transparent, and efficient than ever before. As these advancements continue to unfold, they promise to make supplementation not only more effective but also more aligned with our individual health journeys.

8.3 Personalized Nutrition: The Future of Supplement Plans

Imagine being able to tailor your nutrition plan to the unique blueprint of your body, rather than relying on generic guidelines. Personalized nutrition is reshaping how we approach supplements, offering a more targeted way to support our health. At the heart of this transformation is the integration of DNA-based dietary recommendations. By analyzing your genetic makeup, professionals can determine which nutrients your body needs more of and which ones you might want to avoid. This genetic insight allows for the creation of supplement plans that cater specifically to your biological requirements, enhancing both effectiveness and safety.

Another innovative approach in personalized nutrition is microbiome analysis. The gut is often referred to as the body's second brain, and the balance of bacteria within it can significantly influence your overall health. Through detailed analysis of your microbiome, experts can identify imbalances and recommend specific supplements that promote a healthier gut environment. This tailored supplementation not only helps in optimizing digestion but also boosts immunity and even improves mental health. By understanding the intricacies of your gut flora, you can make informed choices about which probiotics or prebiotics might benefit you most.

The benefits of personalization extend beyond just improved efficacy. When supplements are tailored to your individual needs, there's a noticeable increase in consumer engagement and satisfaction. Knowing that your supplement plan is designed specifically for you fosters a deeper connection to your health regimen. It also reduces the trial-and-error process, where you might otherwise spend time and money on products that don't work for you. Personalized plans mean that every supplement you take has a purpose, aligning with your specific health goals and needs, thus enhancing your overall wellness journey.

Recent technological advancements are making personalized nutrition more accessible than ever. At-home testing kits are becoming a staple for those eager to understand their nutritional deficiencies. These kits allow you to collect samples in the comfort of your home, which are then analyzed to provide insights into your vitamin and mineral levels. This data can guide your supplement choices, ensuring you're addressing any deficiencies effectively. In addition, wearable devices that monitor nutrient levels are entering the market. These gadgets provide real-time feedback on your body's needs, helping you adjust your supplement intake as necessary.

Several companies are leading the charge in personalized nutrition, offering innovative solutions that blend cutting-edge science with user-friendly platforms. Habit is one such company, providing personalized nutrition plans based on a combination of genetic, biometric, and behavioral data. Their approach ensures that each dietary recommendation is backed by comprehensive personal insights. Nutrigenomix offers genetic testing services that delve into how your DNA affects your response to nutrition and exercise. By understanding these genetic influences, they can recommend tailored supplements that maximize your health outcomes.

This shift towards personalization represents a significant evolution in how we perceive and use supplements. No longer confined to one-size-fits-all solutions, personalized nutrition empowers you to take control of your health with precision and confidence. It's about recognizing that your body is unique and deserves a tailored approach to nutrition that reflects your individual needs. Embracing personalized nutrition means stepping into a future where supplements are more than just pills—they're an integral part of a comprehensive strategy for optimal health.

8.4 Innovations in Supplement Delivery: Beyond Pills and Powders

Imagine a world where taking your daily vitamins feels less like gulping down pills and more like enjoying a refreshing drink or applying a discreet patch. This evolving landscape of supplement delivery is reshaping how we consume nutrients, moving beyond the traditional capsules and tablets. Liquid and gel-based formats are gaining traction, offering a smoother, more palatable experience. These formats are not just about ease; they also promise enhanced absorption. When nutrients are suspended in liquid or gel, your body can often absorb them more efficiently than in solid forms. This means you might feel the benefits faster, which is particularly appealing if you're someone who dislikes swallowing pills or is looking for quicker results.

The convenience factor cannot be understated. Dissolvable strips and patches are emerging as game-changers for those with busy lifestyles. A dissolvable strip, similar to a breath mint, can deliver your daily dose of vitamins without needing water. This makes it incredibly simple to get your nutrients on the go, whether you're commuting or traveling. Patches, too, offer a unique advantage. Applied directly to your skin, they provide a slow, steady release of nutrients. This method can ensure more consistent levels of vitamins in your bloodstream, potentially leading to better outcomes. It's a hands-off approach that fits seamlessly into daily life, especially for those who value simplicity and efficiency.

Behind these innovative delivery systems are cutting-edge technologies that are pushing the boundaries of what's possible. Liposomal encapsulation is one such advancement, enhancing the bioavailability of supplements. By encasing nutrients in tiny, fat-like particles called liposomes, this technology helps them bypass the harsh environment of the stomach, reaching the bloodstream more intact. This means that your body can utilize more of the nutrient, making each dose more effective. It's a sophisticated method that aligns with the growing demand for efficient, high-performing supplements.

Several companies are at the forefront of these innovations, setting new standards in the industry. Quicksilver Scientific, for example, is renowned for its liposomal supplements, which offer superior absorption and efficacy. Their products are designed to maximize nutrient delivery, ensuring you get the most out of every dose. OnMi is another brand pushing the envelope with vitamin patches. These patches provide a convenient alternative to oral supplements, ideal for those who prefer a non-ingestible option. By embracing these innovative methods, these companies are meeting consumer demand for products that are both effective and user-friendly.

Incorporating these advanced delivery systems into your supplement routine can transform how you experience nutrition. Whether you choose a fast-acting liquid, a convenient patch, or a cutting-edge liposomal product, the key is to find what fits best with your lifestyle and health goals. As these technologies continue to evolve, they promise to make supplementation not just easier, but more enjoyable and effective. The future of supplements is here, offering options that cater to individual preferences and modern needs.

8.5 Community and Support: Building a Supplement User Network

Imagine walking into a room full of people who share your interests, your questions, and your passion for health and wellness. This is the power of community when it comes to supplement use. Engaging with others who are on a similar path can transform your supplement experience, turning isolation into a shared adventure. By connecting with a community, you gain access to a wealth of shared knowledge and experiences. When someone mentions how a particular supplement improved their energy levels or another shares a cautionary tale about an unexpected reaction, these stories enrich your understanding and guide your choices. Community isn't just about information; it's about the emotional support and encouragement that comes from knowing you're not alone in navigating the often overwhelming world of supplements.

In today's digital age, finding or creating a community is easier than ever. Online platforms like social media groups and forums have become gathering places for supplement enthusiasts. These virtual spaces are buzzing with activity, where members exchange advice, share personal experiences, and pose questions. In a Facebook group dedicated to mental well-being, for example, you might find discussions on which adaptogens have helped others manage stress. On Reddit's supplement subreddit, users dissect scientific studies, breaking down complex information into digestible pieces. These platforms offer a sense of belonging and a space where everyone's voice can be heard, regardless of location. But it's not all online; local health and wellness meetups can also bring people together. These face-to-face interactions foster deeper connections and offer opportunities for hands-on learning, like workshops on making homemade herbal tinctures or guided tours of a local health store.

Communities do more than just share tips and stories; they play a critical role in education and advocacy. Peer reviews and recommendations within these groups often carry more weight than traditional advertising, as they come from real experiences rather than marketing campaigns. When someone in your community gives a thumbs-up to a new supplement brand, it's based on personal results, making it a trusted recommendation. Moreover, communities can rally together to advocate for regulatory changes and transparency in the supplement industry. When a group of passionate individuals raises concerns about misleading labels or unverified claims, they can influence industry standards and push for more stringent regulations. This collective voice empowers consumers and holds companies accountable, driving improvements that benefit everyone.

Successful supplement user communities are thriving across various platforms, illustrating the impact of shared experience. On Reddit's supplement subreddit, members discuss everything from the latest research to personal anecdotes, creating a rich tapestry of information that's both informative and engaging. Facebook groups dedicated to specific health goals, like improving sleep or boosting immunity, provide tailored support where members can dive deep into niche topics. These communities are places of learning, where curiosity and camaraderie fuel a continuous exchange of ideas. Here, members find the motivation they need to stay committed to their health goals, supported by a network that understands their journey.

8.6 Preparing for the Next Wave: Trends to Watch in Supplementation

In recent years, a significant shift has been unfolding in the supplement industry, driven by emerging trends that are reshaping how we think about health and wellness. One of the most compelling developments is the focus on mental health and cognitive enhancement. As the pressures of modern life increase, more individuals are seeking supplements that promise to boost brain function and improve emotional well-being. This has led to a surge in adaptogenic and nootropic supplements, which are designed to enhance cognitive performance and help the body adapt to stress. These products are gaining popularity among students, professionals, and anyone looking to maintain mental clarity in a demanding world.

Consumer preferences are also evolving, with a growing demand for transparency and clean labels. Today's consumers are more informed than ever, and they expect honesty from the brands they trust. They want to know exactly what they're putting into their bodies, without any hidden ingredients or misleading claims. This has prompted many companies to adopt clearer labeling practices and to focus on holistic and integrative health approaches. People are interested in how supplements can fit into a broader lifestyle that includes diet, exercise, and mindfulness. They seek products that not only support specific health goals but also contribute to overall well-being.

The regulatory landscape is responding to these consumer-driven changes with stricter labeling requirements and increased scrutiny of health claims. Authorities are more vigilant in ensuring that the information on supplement labels is accurate and not exaggerated. This shift aims to protect consumers and ensure that they can make informed decisions about their health. Companies are now held to higher standards, which drives innovation and encourages the development of products that truly deliver on their promises.

Industry experts predict several exciting developments on the horizon. One of the most anticipated trends is the expansion of plant-based and vegan supplements. As more people embrace plant-based diets for health, ethical, or environmental reasons, the demand for vegan-friendly supplements is set to rise. These products cater to a growing segment of the population that seeks high-quality nutrition without animal-derived ingredients. Additionally, there is a growing interest in integrating supplements with holistic wellness programs. This approach recognizes that supplements are most effective when used alongside other health practices, such as balanced nutrition, regular physical activity, and mental health support.

As these trends continue to evolve, they will undoubtedly shape the future of supplementation. The industry is moving towards a more transparent, personalized, and integrative approach to health, which promises to empower individuals to take greater control over their well-being. This shift not only reflects changing consumer demands but also represents a broader movement towards a more holistic understanding of health, one that recognizes the complex interplay between mind, body, and environment. As we look ahead, the supplement industry is poised to play a pivotal role in supporting this new paradigm of wellness.

9

Conclusion

As you reach the end of this journey through "Supplements 101," it's important to reflect on the essential insights we've explored together. We've delved into the foundational knowledge necessary to understand supplements, from their definition and purpose to the science behind how they work. By learning about the various types of supplements and their roles in holistic health, you're now equipped to make informed choices that align with your personal wellness goals.

Throughout this book, we have emphasized the importance of making informed decisions. This involves recognizing potential interactions, and integrating supplements safely into your daily life. You've learned strategies for creating personalized supplement plans and how these can be tailored to your unique health needs. This personalized approach allows you to harness the benefits of supplements effectively, ensuring they complement rather than replace a balanced diet.

One of the key takeaways from our discussions is the critical role supplements can play in holistic health. They are not standalone solutions but part of a broader lifestyle that includes nutrition, exercise, and mindfulness. By integrating supplements into your routine, you can support your body's natural functions and enhance your overall well-being. This book has also introduced you to emerging trends such as personalized nutrition and innovative delivery methods, which promise to make supplementation more effective and tailored to individual needs.

Now, it's time to take action. Armed with the knowledge from this book, I encourage you to consult with healthcare professionals to personalize your supplement strategy further. Engage with reputable sources for ongoing learning and connect with communities to share experiences and gain support. Apply the practical tips and strategies we've discussed to enhance your health and wellness confidently.

Remember, the journey to better health is a personal one, and you are capable of making informed decisions that will positively impact your life. With the insights gained from this book, you are well-equipped to navigate the supplement landscape effectively. Trust in your ability to use natural remedies as part of your wellness arsenal. Know that you have the power to achieve your health goals through informed decision-making.

This book stands out as a valuable resource because of its science-backed advice and practical applications. It covers both traditional and emerging topics comprehensively. My commitment to clarity and credibility ensures that you have a reliable guide on your journey toward wellness. By providing this information, I aim to empower you, giving you the confidence to make the best decisions for your health.

As you continue your exploration of the supplement world, I invite you to stay curious and open to new information. Subscribe to health newsletters, follow relevant blogs, or join discussion forums to keep learning. The world of supplements is ever-evolving, and staying informed will only enhance your ability to make choices that benefit your health and well-being.

Thank you for allowing me to be a part of your wellness journey. I hope this book serves as a trusted companion as you explore the healing power of nature and embrace the potential of supplements in your everyday life.

105

Resources

U.S. Food and Drug Administration. (n.d.). *Dietary supplements.* Retrieved from https://www.fda.gov/food/dietary-supplements

Bioavailability of oral vitamins, minerals, and trace elements. (n.d.). *PubMed.* Retrieved from https://pubmed.ncbi.nlm.nih.gov/9150856/

Herbal medicines: Where is the evidence? (n.d.). *PubMed Central (PMC).* Retrieved from https://www.ncbi.nlm.nih.gov/pmc/articles/PMC1127780/

Synthetic vs natural nutrients: Does it matter? (n.d.). *Healthline.* Retrieved from https://www.healthline.com/nutrition/synthetic-vs-natural-nutrients

U.S. Pharmacopeia. (n.d.). *How to read a supplement label | Quality matters.* Retrieved from https://qualitymatters.usp.org/how-read-supplement-label

Healthline. (2024). *11 best vitamin brands in 2024: Healthline's top picks.* Retrieved from https://www.healthline.com/nutrition/best-vitamin-brands

Fullscript. (n.d.). *Easily build supplement plans for optimal health.* Retrieved from https://fullscript.com/

Tricks of the trade: Are supplement companies playing you for a fool? (n.d.). *Center for Science in the Public Interest (CSPI).* Retrieved from https://www.cspinet.org/article/tricks-trade-are-supplement-companies-playing-you-fool

Office of Dietary Supplements. (n.d.). *Nutrient recommendations and databases.* Retrieved from https://ods.od.nih.gov/HealthInformation/nutrientrecommendations.aspx

Dietary supplements: Benefits, side effects, risks, and outlook. (n.d.). *Healthline.* Retrieved from https://www.healthline.com/health/nutrition/dietary-supplements

Mayo Clinic. (n.d.). *St. John's wort.* Retrieved from https://www.mayoclinic.org/drugs-supplements-st-johns-wort/art-20362212

Healthline. (n.d.). *Supplements during pregnancy: What's safe and what's not.* Retrieved from https://www.healthline.com/nutrition/supplements-during-pregnancy

Office of Dietary Supplements. (n.d.). *Omega-3 fatty acids - Health professional fact sheet.* Retrieved from https://ods.od.nih.gov/factsheets/Omega3FattyAcids-HealthProfessional/

Cheng, S. (2019, February 4). *The best time of day to take common nutritional supplements. The Washington Post.* Retrieved from https://www.washingtonpost.com/lifestyle/wellness/morning-or-night-with-food-or-without-answers-to-your-questions-about-taking-supplements/2019/02/04/5fcec02a-2577-11e9-81fd-b7b05d5bed90_story.html

Transportation Security Administration (TSA). (n.d.). *Supplements.* Retrieved from https://www.tsa.gov/travel/security-screening/whatcanibring/items/supplements

Swolverine. (n.d.). *Joint health supplement stack for athletes.* Retrieved from https://swolverine.com/products/joint-health

Healthline. (n.d.). *CoQ10 (coenzyme Q10) dosage.* Retrieved from https://www.healthline.com/nutrition/coq10-dosage

NutraIngredients. (2024). *Combatting stress: Efficacy and safety of Rhodiola rosea and Ashwagandha reviewed.* Retrieved from https://www.nutraingredients.com/Article/2024/02/22/Combatting-stress-Efficacy-and-safety-of-Rhodiola-rosea-and-Ashwagandha-reviewed

The effect of melatonin, magnesium, and zinc on primary insomnia.

(n.d.). *PubMed.* Retrieved from https://pubmed.ncbi.nlm.nih.gov/212 26679/

Mayo Clinic. (n.d.). *Probiotics and prebiotics: What you should know.* Retrieved from https://www.mayoclinic.org/healthy-lifestyle/nutriti on-and-healthy-eating/expert-answers/probiotics/faq-20058065

National Institutes of Health, Office of Dietary Supplements. (n.d.). *Omega-3 fatty acids: Health professional fact sheet.* Retrieved from https://ods.od.nih.gov/factsheets/Omega3FattyAcids-HealthProfess ional/

Frontiers in Nutrition. (2023). Advances and trends in nutraceutical and functional plant research. *Frontiers in Nutrition.* Retrieved from https://www.frontiersin.org/journals/nutrition/articles/10.3389/fn ut.2023.1168826/full

Stough, C., Lloyd, J., Clarke, J., Downey, L. A., Hutchison, C. W., Rodgers, T., & Nathan, P. J. (2001). Effects of a standardized *Bacopa monnieri* extract on cognitive performance in healthy human subjects. *Journal of Psychopharmacology, 15*(4), 374–384. Retrieved from https://w ww.ncbi.nlm.nih.gov/pmc/articles/PMC3153866/

Verdin, E. (2022). The role of NAD+ in regenerative medicine. *Frontiers in Aging Neuroscience, 14,* 9512238. Retrieved from https://w ww.ncbi.nlm.nih.gov/pmc/articles/PMC9512238/

American Medical Association. (2023). What doctors wish patients knew about vitamins and supplements. Retrieved from https://www.a ma-assn.org/delivering-care/public-health/what-doctors-wish-patie nts-knew-about-vitamins-and-supplements

GoodRx Health. (n.d.). My experience with berberine for weight loss. Retrieved from https://www.goodrx.com/conditions/weight-loss/m y-experience-with-berberine

Human Tonik. (n.d.). Dave Asprey supplements: What does he take? Retrieved from https://humantonik.com/dave-asprey-supplements/

Healthline. (2023). 12 powerful Ayurvedic herbs and spices with health benefits. Retrieved from https://www.healthline.com/nutritio n/ayurvedic-herbs

Sustainable Jungle. (n.d.). 9 sustainable supplements & vitamins for a healthier you. Retrieved from https://www.sustainablejungle.com/ sustainable-supplements-vitamins/

Supplement Factory UK. (2023). Artificial intelligence in supplement formulations: A new era or a passing fad? Retrieved from https://sup plementfactoryuk.com/blog/2023/08/artificial-intelligence-in-suppl ement-formulations-a-new-era-or-a-passing-fad/

Reports and Data. (n.d.). Top 10 companies in the personalized nutrition industry. Retrieved from https://www.reportsanddata.com/ blog/top-companies-in-the-personalized-nutrition-industry

Nutritional Outlook. (n.d.). Innovative new delivery systems for dietary supplements. Retrieved from https://www.nutritionaloutlook. com/view/delivery-systems-take-brave-new-formats